SKID ROAD

SKID
ROAD

■ ■ ■ ■ ■ ■ ■ ■ ■

ON THE FRONTIER

OF HEALTH AND HOMELESSNESS

IN AN AMERICAN CITY

Josephine Ensign

Johns Hopkins University Press

BALTIMORE

© 2021 Johns Hopkins University Press
All rights reserved. Published 2021
Printed in the United States of America on acid-free paper
2 4 6 8 9 7 5 3 1

Johns Hopkins University Press
2715 North Charles Street
Baltimore, Maryland 21218-4363
www.press.jhu.edu

Library of Congress Cataloging-in-Publication Data
Names: Ensign, Josephine, author.
Title: Skid Road : on the frontier of health and homelessness
in an American city / Josephine Ensign.
Description: Baltimore : Johns Hopkins University Press, [2021]
Includes bibliographical references and index.
Identifiers: LCCN 2020015931
ISBN 9781421440132 (hardcover)
ISBN 9781421440149 (ebook)
Subjects:
LCSH: Homelessness—Washington (State)—Seattle—History. |
Homeless persons—Health and hygiene—Washington (State)—
Seattle—History. | Mentally ill homeless persons—Washington
(State)—Seattle—History. | Skid row—Washington (State)—
Seattle—History.
Classification: LCC HV4506.S43 E57 2021
DDC 362.1086/942—dc23
LC record available at https://lccn.loc.gov/2020015931

A catalog record for this book is available from the British Library.

*Special discounts are available for bulk purchases of this book. For more
information, please contact Special Sales at specialsales@jh.edu.*

Johns Hopkins University Press uses environmentally friendly book
materials, including recycled text paper that is composed of at least
30 percent post-consumer waste, whenever possible.

Typeset in Chaparral Pro by Amy Ruth Buchanan/3rd sister design.

For Peter

Every day we tread

over Chief Sealth's legacy

his prophetic words,

"At night, when the streets

. . . will be silent and you think

them deserted,

they will throng

with the returning hosts

that once filled them

and still love this beautiful land."

We are not alone

save for his people

we are all immigrants here

waiter, teacher

artist, worker, nurse

we belong

all of us belong

Seattle is a house

we all need to afford.

—Claudia Castro Luna, "Seattle's Poem"

CONTENTS

SKID ROAD

ONE WOMAN'S SEATTLE

At the foot of the hills, between the office buildings
and the bay, lies a narrow strip of land:
here on the waterfront Seattle's history and
Seattle's future meet and merge.
—Murray Morgan,
Skid Road: An Informal Portrait of Seattle

The hills are so steep in downtown Seattle that many of the side-walks have horizontal raised ridges, like logs laid down cross-wise, to keep people from tumbling down, especially when it rains.[1] It is raining on this November day as I walk down Yesler Way from Harborview Medical Center toward the oldest part of Seattle: Pioneer Square.

Yesler Way, once called Mill Street as well as Skid Road, is one of Seattle's first roads, made by white pioneers and Native Americans who worked for Seattle's earliest entrepreneur, Henry Yesler. In the early 1850s, his workers cut the towering old-growth fir and cedar trees thickly lining the hills around the small village on the banks of Puget Sound. The rough road was lined with partially buried logs—skids—which were laid across the mud road at seven-foot intervals to allow the men to roll the freshly cut trees down the steep hill to Yesler's sawmill on the waterfront. The skids were kept lubricated by a low-paid and nimble logger—a greaser—who ran ahead of the tumbling logs, splashing the skids with salmon oil from a bucket. Early visitors joked that they could smell Seattle before they could see it due to the pungent, rancid fish odor emanating from the settlement.

The odor of Seattle has changed considerably from those early days, as, of course, has the entire city. On this rainy November day, walking down Skid Road—Yesler Way—toward the waterfront, I smell car, truck, and earth-moving equipment exhaust mixed with the tang of saltwater carried on the wind from Puget Sound, part of the Salish Sea. I am on my way to the Chief Seattle Club located in the heart of Pioneer Square. At the bottom of the hill, I stop at the paved, wedge-shaped Pioneer Square park with its Victorian era iron pergola, its elegant but now sealed-off underground public restrooms, and its Tlingit sixty-foot-tall cedar Chief-of-All-Women totem pole. This is the land where Yesler's sawmill stood. I notice an art installation that I had previously overlooked, thinking it was merely public signage. Next to a bronze bust of Chief Sealth, for whom Seattle is named, is *Day/Night* by Cheyenne Arapaho artist Hachivi Edgar Heap of Birds. It consists of two ceramic panels covered in green dollar signs and crosses, with bold black text in both Coast Salish and English that states, "Chief Seattle now the streets are our home." The installation is dedicated to Seattle's Native American homeless people, of which there are a disproportionate number.

Across Yesler Way from the park is the Chief Seattle Club, which provides food, day shelter, an arts program, and healthcare to Seattle's Indigenous homeless adult population. I am scheduled to be there today as the faculty nurse preceptor for a group of university health science students providing basic foot care. As I walk toward the Chief Seattle Club, I pass through another small park, Fortson Square, which has a public art installation of concrete building ruins—including a fallen and fractured Corinthian column—and bits of poetry in the bricks paving the ground. Glancing down, I notice that one of the bricks, partially covered in cedar chips, is inscribed with "Skid Road." Other bricks, spaced apart and running downhill, read, "We are proud people and we survive." Even in the steady drizzle, this area is thronged with people dressed in stained, soggy clothing sitting on the concrete ruins. A woman is wrapped in a bright red blanket. They all appear to be patiently, or resignedly, waiting for something. An older man with a bandaged lower leg, shuffling slowly with a walker, stops to ask me where the Lazarus Center is. I tell him it is just up ahead, next door to the Chief Seattle Club.

In the foot clinic that day, we see a gray-haired man from a Coast Salish tribe, who tells us he was a logger in Alaska for six years back in the 1980s. He describes the repeated injuries he sustained from the work, especially to his lower legs. He had surgery at Harborview Medical Center on one leg to repair a "nasty fracture" and had two pins put in the ankle. Harborview is the Level I trauma center for Washington, Alaska, Montana, and Idaho—a land mass close to 250,000 square kilometers—and is the King County hospital with a mission of providing quality healthcare to indigent, homeless, mentally ill, incarcerated, and growing refugee and immigrant populations. This former logger now has diabetes, uses a walker, and lives in an emergency shelter across the street, with his healthcare coming from Harborview and the Indian Health Board. Later that day, I meet another older man with long salt-and-pepper hair tied back by a red bandanna. In the arts and crafts room, he proudly shows me the intricately carved pipes he makes out of deer antlers he finds scattered around his reservation on the nearby Olympic Peninsula. He sells the pipes to tourists along the Seattle waterfront and in Pioneer Square near its numerous restaurants and bars.

"These pipes are more popular now that weed is legal here," he tells me with a laugh.

■ ■ ■

Seattle is my adopted hometown. Like many other people, I moved here from a much older, more problem-plagued city in search of greater opportunities and a better quality of life—and as an escape from my past. The city where I was living in the early 1990s, Baltimore, had the highest murder rate in the country, along with one of the highest high school drop-out rates. I am a nurse and researcher who works with homeless people. In Baltimore, the homeless teens I worked with told me things like, "Even if I live to be a hundred, which I won't, I'll always be sad." The burned and boarded-up rowhouses in the area where I worked and lived were often on dead-end streets. When my car broke down one evening after work, no towing company wanted to send a truck because it was too dangerous. A tow truck did eventually show up, but the driver brandished a shotgun. I was burned-out on trying to nudge things there in a better direction. For me at the time, that meant moving west to the much younger, more progressive—and much more hopeful—city of Seattle.

When this book is published in 2021, I will have lived and worked in Seattle for twenty-seven years. It is the longest I have ever lived in one place, and Seattle has proven to be a good city for me personally and professionally. Of course, Seattle is not without its problems, including homelessness and its attendant ills. Seattle now has the third-highest number of homeless people in the United States, behind New York and Los Angeles. Per capita, Seattle likely has the highest rate of homelessness in the country. The King County Medical Examiner's Office reports on the number of people it investigates who die while homeless; there were 1,056 deaths between 2012 and the end of 2019, and there was a record number of 196 deaths of homeless people in

2018.[2] Compared with the deaths for the housed population, homeless people who die in King County (Seattle is the official seat of King County) are much younger and more likely to be people of color, including Native Americans. Many die outside from hypothermia or complications of chronic diseases. Most of the younger homeless people die of drug overdoses and suicide. A large number of homeless people have an underlying mental illness, including depression, post-traumatic stress disorder, and schizophrenia. It is important to point out that significant traumas, including childhood traumas, often precede and complicate the experience of homelessness. And the chaos, insecurity, and exposure to violence that accompany homelessness exacerbate preexisting mental and physical health problems. The King County Board of Health declared homelessness a public health disaster in the early fall of 2018.

How do we reconcile the fact that Seattle is both a progressive, hopeful city and a place in which homelessness is such a large, growing, and deeply entrenched problem? Is it, as many critics claim, precisely because of our progressive politics and so many "bleeding-heart liberals" that people are attracted to the city and then stay stuck in homelessness and poverty? Or is it, as other people say, because of the greediness of large Seattle-based corporations and our city's concessions—selling out—to them? This book is a result of my quest to know more about Seattle's history regarding health and homelessness, my desire to know the roots of our current situation in order to help inform policy and advocacy solutions.

■ ■ ■

I am a southerner from the capital of the Confederacy, Richmond, Virginia. Southerners are known for having a strong sense of place. By "place," I mean both geography and "knowing one's place" within the rigid lines of race, class, and gender. And "place" also refers to a physical location layered with a multiplicity of narratives, with hauntings of individual and collective—often deeply traumatic and suppressed—stories. Every location has these aspects to some degree if we are willing to stop, wait, and listen. The historian Coll Thrush aptly terms these "place-stories" or "place-bound histories in urban space." He asks, "Can remnants of past societies—ruins, ecological footprints, artifacts—'speak' in active ways for the histories they represent?"[3] He answers in the affirmative and backs this up with volumes of evidence, much of it focused on the histories of Indigenous Seattle.[4] I agree with Thrush, and I have applied his concept of place-stories in the research and writing of this book.

In this book, a work of narrative history, I explore the intersection of safety-net healthcare and homelessness in Seattle, Washington. My intention is to deepen our understanding of the historical roots of poverty and homelessness, trauma and resilience, and the roles of charity and safety-net healthcare and public policy in Seattle–King County. I am interested in how a large, relatively young, socially progressive urban area like Seattle responds to the health and social needs of people marginalized by poverty and homelessness.

More than a nod of acknowledgment is due for the influence of the now-classic book by Murray Morgan, *Skid Road: An Informal Portrait of Seattle*, first published in 1951. In his preface, titled "One Man's Seattle," Morgan states that he aimed to write the history of "Seattle from the bottom up." For Morgan, the "bottom" meant the people "who weren't quite respectable but helped build the great city of the Northwest."[5] He includes stories of people like Seattle's first physician, David "Doc" Maynard, and other "men who dreamed the wrong dreams."[6] My aim with my *Skid Road* is to dig even deeper through the layers of Seattle's history—past its leaders and prominent people, respectable or not (and not just men)—to the stories of the overlooked and unheard people living and dying at the margins. Their stories (often, mere fragments of stories), their lives and deaths, are not included in official histories of most places, including Seattle. The marginalized and the margins in which they are located in many ways define, or literally frame, our collective lives. And, akin to the fact that the origins of a human being deeply influence but do not define their personality and future trajectory, the origins of a city resonate through time and leave their tracings.

■ ■ ■

Clinging to steep hills at one of the far western edges of the North American continent, with abundant rainfall, a deep inland sea rich with life, and trees of enormous proportion, Seattle was a latecomer among cities in the United States. Although visited by fur trappers associated with England's Hudson's Bay Company beginning in the 1700s, Seattle was not settled by European American pioneers until 1852.[7] It was officially incorporated as a city in 1869, four years after the end of the US Civil War and the year that the first transcontinental railroad was completed, with its western terminus in San Francisco.

Indigenous peoples have lived on this land for thousands and likely tens of thousands of years. Recently, a series of bare human footprints from two adults and a child were found on the tide line of a Canadian island in the Salish Sea not far from Seattle.[8] The footprints were carbon-dated at 13,000 years old. These are the oldest human footprints found to date in North America and support the theory that the first humans to come to the Americas migrated from northeastern Asia to the Pacific Northwest about 16,000 years ago by sea along the "kelp highway" and not solely by land across the Bering Strait. The subsequent Pacific Northwest Indigenous tribes, including the Duwamish of the land that became the city of Seattle and of which Seattle, also referred to as Sealth, was chief, developed their languages, medicine, arts, crafts, and other aspects of culture long before the first white man ever visited, hunted, logged, doctored, stayed to live—or became homeless—in the area.

Counties are the oldest local government entities in the Pacific Northwest, and King County was formed by the Oregon territorial legislature in late December 1852. Washington was separated from Oregon in March 1853. From its early days, the government of Seattle–King County has been responsible for supporting indigents, paupers, and ill, insane, and homeless people living in the county. Beginning in 1854 with the discovery of the area's first homeless "insane pauper," which was followed by the 1877 establishment of the King County Poor Farm along the Duwamish River and the transformation of a former opium-smuggling boat into a Seattle waterfront emergency hospital, through the 1931 opening of Harborview Hospital, to the current array of regional trauma care and community-based services of the Harborview Medical Center, the leaders and residents of Seattle–King County have wrestled with ways to fulfill and pay for this public mandate and mission.

The research for this book included documents, newspaper articles, letters, and photographs in libraries and in government and hospital archives. From 2014 to 2017, I did ethnographic immersion and observations in the public spaces of Pioneer Square and the University District, around homeless encampments throughout Seattle, near Harborview Medical Center, and in public areas near other safety-net healthcare service sites in Seattle–King County. In addition, I conducted a series of thirty-six professionally audio- and video-recorded oral histories with people working and living at the intersection of health and homelessness in King County. Their stories, along with findings from the ethnographic research, are woven into the fabric of this book, mainly in later chapters. Present-day King County includes Puget Sound islands like Vashon and Bainbridge and large swaths of the Cascade mountains to the east of Seattle.

While homelessness occurs throughout King County, the largest concentration is in the city of Seattle. Therefore, my focus in this book is on health and homelessness in that city.

■ ■ ■

Am I my brother's keeper? Are we our brothers' and sisters' keepers? These are my questions while walking the Seattle waterfront on a blazingly sunny late July afternoon in 2018. I am in search of the most likely coordinates for the location along the shoreline where Seattle's first homeless person, the first official "insane pauper," was found 164 years ago. In late 1854, Seattle had fewer than 50 non-Indigenous residents, and most of them were scattered on homesteads outside of town. In 2018, the city of Seattle had a population of more than 730,000 people, with close to 4 million living in the Seattle metropolitan area.

The King County Point-in-Time Count on January 26, 2018, found an estimated 8,600 homeless people in the city of Seattle and a total of 12,112 people experiencing homelessness in all of King County. But those numbers were only the people experiencing literal homelessness, meaning they were living on the streets, in encampments or vehicles, or in emergency shelters. The count did not include the significant number of "hidden" homeless people, especially young people and families with young children, who were doubled up with friends, or living in and out of cheap hotels (often with pimps), or otherwise with no stable, safe place to live. The best approach to the provision and financing of care for Seattle's homeless people continues to confound the residents of King County.

As I walk north along the boardwalk from the end of Skid Road (Yesler Way), dodging throngs of camera-wielding tourists, passing shops still displaying shrunken heads and human skeletons next to piles of carved wooden "Indian totem poles," I search for the most likely location along the shoreline where residents of Seattle found the man destined to become the city's first homeless person.

This can never be proven definitively, but by triangulating multiple sources of evidence, I have concluded that Seattle's first homeless person most likely lived where the Seattle Marriott Waterfront Hotel now stands at the corner of Lenora Street and Alaskan Way. The hotel is an eight-story, shiny steel and glass building near the World Trade Center. As I stand on the boardwalk looking at the hotel, a loud freight train moves on tracks just behind the building. The hill climbs gently here, and the towering office buildings and new high-rise condominiums of Belltown jostle for space. Up the hill to the right are the sprawling buildings of the Pike Place Market. Its kitschy flying-fish tourist act vies for attention along with the ghost of a Native princess, the daughter of Chief Seattle, who once lived in a wood shack at this location. Underneath the raised Alaskan Way Viaduct (since torn down in favor of an underground tunnel for through traffic), I see a line of homeless encampments with tents, blue tarps, and piles of trash cascading down the hillside.

Turning to take in the water view from this spot, I see rust-red crabs on the barnacle-encrusted rocks, egg-yolk jellyfish, and beds of undulating giant sea kelp. Squawking seagulls bob on the waves. There is a heavy salt smell mixed with hot creosote from the wharf pilings. And—ah yes—there is the strong smell of fish from the salmon and clam fry shack on the wharf beside me. The beautiful snow-capped giants of Mount Rainier to the south and Mount Olympus to the west are both visible from here.

Looking more closely at the boardwalk area around me, I notice the figure of a young, deeply tanned man lying inside a long cardboard box; his booted feet stick out one end and his head out the other. His face is partially covered with a dirty blue baseball cap. He is lying against a concrete barrier, partially shaded. I know he is sleeping and not unconscious or dead from a drug overdose because I watch long enough to see him move the position of his cap. In front of him, next to a Starbucks paper cup for collecting spare change, is a handwritten cardboard sign: Homeless, Please Help.

Am I my brother's keeper?

Stand beside me now at the intersection of Lenora Street and Alaskan Way on the Seattle waterfront, the waves of the Salish Sea lapping beneath the boardwalk at our feet. Let us look back in time, imagine these place-stories, and listen for the lessons they can teach us today.

1

BROTHER'S KEEPER

In a pioneer community like Seattle no one knew
what to do with an insane pauper.

—Murray Morgan, *Skid Road: An Informal Portrait of Seattle*

Sleet slashed horizontally across the beach and crusted piles of seaweed, kelp, and driftwood on the high tide line; it worried its way through the flaps of a tattered canvas tent nestled between charred tree stumps and onto the muddy rag-wrapped feet of the shivering man lying inside. Wood smoke, mixed with the salt of the inland sea, fir sap, and rotting shellfish, accompanied the hard wind.

Late December 1854 in Seattle was relentlessly cold and wet. The man's tent was the only such structure on this stretch of shoreline along the northern edge of the pioneer settlement. The land had been newly claimed by William Bell but was known to both white settlers and Indigenous people by its Coast Salish name, Babaqwab (Little Prairie), which referred to its stretches of low-growing, berry-producing salal.[1] Piles of clam shells surrounded cedar longhouses built by the Native people: the beach here was rich with butter clams and had long served as an Indigenous seafood-processing area.

The tent dweller was Edward Moore, a thirty-two-year-old sailor from Worcester County, Massachusetts, who had stayed behind in Seattle—or was left behind—by his ship's captain. Perhaps he drank too much even by drunken sailor standards, although there is no record of that. What is known is that he had been living in his makeshift tent for months, living off raw shellfish he foraged and being cared for after a fashion by the Coast Salish people who lived nearby.

Soon after this December day, Edward Moore was deemed by the white pioneer leaders of Seattle to be insane and incapable of taking care of himself. They likely found him in his tent, unable to walk, and carried him along the frozen muddy beach at low tide to the town's one rooming house. There was no hospital. Upon unwrapping the rags covering Moore's feet, it was discovered that he had severe frostbite. The town's first doctor, David Swinson Maynard, promptly amputated most of Moore's toes with an ax. This was, after all, a frontier logging town where medical care was scarce and sharp axes were plentiful. Doc Maynard may have sterilized the ax with the whiskey he was fond of drinking. Moore survived this primitive surgery and was cared for by Doc Maynard; Maynard's second wife and Seattle's first nurse, Catherine; and the German immigrant innkeeper, David Maurer. Edward Moore was King County's first official homeless person. What became of Moore, how the residents and leaders of the nascent town of Seattle dealt with him, and the poignant story of his final days echo lessons and dilemmas that are with us still.

■ ■ ■

The village of Seattle was barely two years old and consisted of fewer than a dozen log and wood-frame houses scattered along the shore just south of where Moore was found. The first population census of King County in 1853—a census that excluded Native people, British, French, and others deemed non-US citizens—found 170 inhabitants. King County at the time extended to include the entire Olympic Peninsula. The immediate Seattle area had at most 50 residents.

Seattle was built on an eight-acre isthmus of marshy land near the mouth of the Duwamish River where it enters Puget Sound. The Indigenous peoples had long used this area as a landing place and fishing camp and called it Sdidelalic, translated as Little Crossing-Over Point. The white settlers called the area either "the Point" or "the Sag" in the early years of its existence. The town was originally registered as Duwamps before the townsfolk, led by Doc Maynard, countered with the name Seattle in honor of his friend Chief Seattle, who had led him to this location and who helped the early settlers survive.[2] At high tide the town was an island, but the low-lying marsh around it was being filled by piles of sawdust from Henry Yesler's steam-powered sawmill.

The sawmill was the area's only industry, and Yesler employed almost all available male settlers and a considerable number of Indigenous men. Since Yesler's mill was established in March 1853, it had been eating through the thick stands of fir and cedar surrounding the fledgling town. The milled lumber was shipped to the gold rush boomtown of San Francisco, and some lumber was used by local settlers to replace their original rough-hewn log cabins. Yesler gave cast-off lumber scraps to local Native people to build small houses along the beach in place of their traditional large cedar longhouses or their more temporary beach shelters made of woven cattails. The cookhouse at Yesler's sawmill was the center of town activities, serving as the early courthouse, church, and saloon, as well as a place to feed and sometimes house the loggers. It was a twenty-five-foot square log cabin with a large fireplace and a covered porch.[3] Yesler's cookhouse was likely where the townsfolk gathered in late December 1854 to discuss what to do with Edward Moore.

The residents of Seattle knew of Moore before he was found half frozen on the beach, as he had become a wandering destitute fixture in the pioneer town. After the crude amputation of Moore's frozen toes, Doc Maynard and his wife, Catherine, took him into their home to care for this "stranger, and insane besides."[4] The Maynards, along with David Maurer who had just opened a small lodging house across Front Street (now First Avenue) from the Maynards' home, cared for Moore for four months. Accounts reveal that together they helped restore Moore's physical health to a large extent, but not his mental health. Physically, Moore was "crippled," presumably a result of the frostbite and amputation of his toes.

■ ■ ■

Who is responsible for paupers, for insane people, for homeless people? Besides the moral imperative to assist people less fortunate, there have long been legal imperatives directed at both the family and public levels. The pioneer settlers of what became Washington State carried the Poor Laws with them across the prairies from places like New England and the Midwest. These Poor Laws were state, or in this case territory, laws originally derived from the sixteenth-century Elizabethan English Poor Laws adopted by the early American colonies.

The English Poor Laws began with the Vagabond and Beggars Act of 1494, which called for all male and female vagabonds and beggars to be put in the stocks for three days and nights, given only bread and water, and then "warned out"—admonished to return to the "hundred" where they were born or last lived. Each hundred, or town parish tied to the church, was responsible for the poor within its jurisdiction. Vagabond and beggar repeat offenders could be—and were—executed.[5] These Poor Laws were expanded through the passage of the Act for the Punishment of Sturdy Vagabonds and Beggars in 1536, which in turn became the Elizabethan Poor Laws codified in 1597–1598 and signed by the Parliament in 1601 as the Act for the Relief of the Poor. For the first time in England, the state, and not the church, was responsible for management of the poor, including the levying of parish-based taxes to pay for poor relief.[6]

The "warned-out" portion of the older law was extended under the Elizabethan Poor Laws and became known as the Act of Settlement, which banned the poor from moving anywhere outside their own parish, even if they were in search of work. This severely limited the geographic and socioeconomic mobility of the poor.[7] It is worth noting that these laws were made by the landed gentry, who had a vested interest in maintaining a pool of local laboring poor people to perform low-paying, dangerous, and unpleasant work.

The Elizabethan Poor Laws established the duty to support, mandating that the primary responsibility for the care and support of a poor person was that person's family. They stipulated the rule of three generations, meaning that the pauper's parents, grandparents, and children were morally and legally responsible for the care of "their own." If the poor person's family either did not exist or could not support their family member, the local parish could auction off the care of the pauper to the highest bidder at a public auction—a thinly veiled version of slavery. A poor person receiving parish support was required to wear a branding on their clothing that identified and literally and figuratively stigmatized them as a charity case. Able-bodied or "sturdy" paupers—as compared with the "impotent poor" who could not work—were regularly rounded up and shipped off to the increasing number of English colonies around the world, including the colonies in America.

The Virginia Colony at Jamestown petitioned the London

Common Council to send a hundred poor and vagabond children who "lie in the streets . . . having no place of abode." In February 1618, the council rounded up and shipped to Jamestown seventy-five boys and twenty-five girls as young as eight years old. None of the children had been convicted of any crime in the London court system, but the council transported them as punishment for being vagrant and "running wild in the streets."[8] Six years later, the records show, only two of these children survived in the Virginia Colony.[9] The rest of the children likely died of the rampant malaria that afflicted the residents of Jamestown, which was built on a swamp.

David Hitchcock, an English social historian, states, "Christian charity and proper punishment were delicately connected in English culture."[10] He terms the banishment of an increasing number of paupers throughout England "welfare colonialism." In England, it was thought that welfare colonialism combined with some level of relief at home for the "deserving poor" would contribute to the quelling of any possible class rebellions and revolutions. Indeed, this approach may have contributed to the fact that England did not undergo the same level of class-based revolutions as those that occurred throughout Europe, especially in 1848.

The first governor of the Massachusetts Bay Colony, the Puritan and wealthy landholder John Winthrop, wrote the lay sermon *A Modell of Christian Charity* in 1630, in which he set forth his vision of the new "City on the Hill" in America. In this sermon, likely written as he sailed from England for what would become Boston, Winthrop made clear that he did not want a social transformation in America, only a spiritual one. He wrote that "God Almighty in His most holy and wise providence hath so dispensed the conditions of mankind, as in all times, some must be rich, some poor." He admonished the rich not to "eat up" the poor, and the poor not to "rise up against and shake off their yoke."[11] Poor people were to be pitied and given direct aid by those better off, and these good works would lead to salvation for the person bestowing charity.

The early American Poor Laws continued variations of the Elizabethan Poor Laws, including the Act of Settlement and the warning out or "passing on" of poor people considered to be outsiders to a parish or county. This has been described as the guiding principle of "help thy neighbor and expel the stranger."[12] States, including Delaware, New Jersey, and Maryland, mandated that recipients of public charity be branded—such as wearing on the left arm a red cloth band with the name of the county from which the pauper was receiving aid.[13]

In the late eighteenth and early nineteenth centuries in the expanding US states and territories, paupers continued to be denied political, civil, and social rights. Poverty was considered an individual and not a societal or economic system failure. The Poor Laws supported the view of poverty as a crime, especially for the "undeserving poor," a category that included any pauper, no matter their age, gender, or condition, deemed by the authorities as able to perform some type of work. Because the "distracted" (an early American term for insanity) and "idiots" were so often poor or vulnerable to exploitation, they were considered "deserving poor" along with the elderly, widows, orphans, and blind people.[14] Children were not excluded from the work requirement and were auctioned off and literally "farmed out" as workers, especially into the expanding American frontier lands. States with seaports allowed the forcing of male paupers to become sailors—a high-risk and low-paying job. Massachusetts made it a crime for a shipmaster to transport and leave a pauper in another location—and, indeed, most states made it a crime for anyone to knowingly leave a pauper outside their home county.[15]

The duty of support by family members was carried over from the Elizabethan Poor Laws. Many states expanded on this in the early 1800s to include grandchildren and siblings in the moral and legal duty to financially support a poor family member.[16] The Act of Settlement was widely adopted and included the stipulation that counties be reimbursed by a pauper's "home" county for any costs of support, including medical care, rendered while the pauper was within its jurisdiction.

The Legislative Assembly of the Territory of Washington passed An Act Relating to the Support of the Poor on May 1, 1854.[17] This original Poor Law stayed as the law in Washington State with only minor amendments well into the twentieth century. Section 1 of the law stipulated that the boards of the counties in the territory should be "vested with the superintendence of the poor in their respective counties." Poor people were defined as anyone "who shall be unable to earn a livelihood in consequence of bodily infirmity, idiocy, lunacy or other cause." It was this Poor Law that the leaders of King County consulted when deciding what to do with Edward Moore, who, because of both his mental and now permanent physical disabilities, was a "deserving" pauper living in their midst.

Despite whatever mental illness Moore had, he was lucid enough to tell his various doctors and caregivers where he was from—Worcester County, Massachusetts—and that he had a wife and children who lived there. They also documented how long he had resided in Seattle–King County—less than six months until he was found half frozen on the Seattle beach. They decided from this information that he was not a resident of King County. The Poor Laws of Washington Territory at that time stipulated a minimum continuous stay of six months in order for a person to establish residency. The residency requirement was increased to twelve months as the territory became more settled and then became Washington State. However, section 6 of the original Poor Law mandated that county officials provide "board, nursing, and medical aid" for any nonresident pauper falling ill while in their county—and, if necessary, provide for the cost of a proper burial.[18]

■ ■ ■

In May 1855, the leaders of Seattle transferred Edward Moore fifty miles south to the then much larger town of Steilacoom to be cared for by physician Matthew P. Burns. Burns gave Doc Maynard a receipt for Moore, "an insane and crippled man, a stranger without acquaintance or friends."[19] It is likely that Steilacoom was considered a safer place to house Moore during the ongoing skirmishes with local Indigenous tribes that were occurring in the region. Steilacoom was a larger and more established settlement than Seattle. Fort Steilacoom was there, which housed a unit of the US Army formed to defend early white settlers from Native people and to establish America's manifest destiny claim on land still marginally occupied and claimed by England. Fort Steilacoom would become in 1871 Western State Hospital, Washington's first public insane asylum, which continues in operation, albeit problematically, at the same location today.

During the time that the residents of Seattle–King County were working through what to do about the plight of Edward Moore, the understanding and medical treatment of mental illness in the United States was undergoing radical change. Up until the beginning of the nineteenth century in Europe and America, mental and physical ailments were lumped together and largely attributed to spiritual causes and were treated accordingly. Heroic measures, including bloodletting, purging, and blistering, were the main treatments for mental illness at that time. These heroic measures were used in conjunction with restraint, including shackles, cuffs, and straitjackets, and locking patients in bare jail cells when families could no longer care for the person or when no family existed. Patients deemed insane were often tranquilized with the liberal use of opiates, especially in the form of morphine.[20] Then, beginning with advances in France and England, which soon spread to New England, moral treatment started to take hold.

French physician Philippe Pinel is credited with developing this new approach to mental illness treatment and with coining the term *traitement moral*, which was mistranslated into English (especially once it reached pious New England) as "morality" instead of the French meaning of the word as it was used then, "well-being" or "morale," as in good spirits.[21] Pinel and other proponents of moral treatment advocated for the release of lunatics from chains and for them to live in quiet places with regimented but kindly discipline. For the first time, mental health experts believed that it was essential to remove patients from the environment that had contributed—if not outright caused—their maladies. Hence, the terms "asylum" and "retreat" began to be synonymous with the insane hospital. Proponents of moral care advocated for a "meticulously sane" environment for the ideal asylum, with a strict daily routine, employment of some type of outdoor exercise, and intellectual stimulation through on-site libraries and lecture series.[22]

This sort of ideal care for the mentally ill was, of course, not available in or near Seattle in the 1850s while the residents were figuring out what to do with Moore. Seattle and, indeed, the entire Washington Territory at the time had no specific provisions or places for insane people. Ironically, and probably known to medical people like Doc Maynard, Massachusetts and specifically Worcester County where Edward Moore was from, had one of the nation's best insane asylums. In 1833, Massachusetts had opened the country's first state-supported public mental hospital, the Worcester Insane Asylum.[23] It was built in the architectural style of the panopticon devised by the English philosopher and social reformer Jeremy Bentham.[24] Massachusetts was also home to the leading mental illness treatment reformer of the time, an intrepid woman who would make her way out west to Washington Territory: Dorothea Dix.

Starting in 1830 with her investigative reporting on the deplorable conditions of inmates at a Cambridge, Massachusetts, jail, Dix spread her advocacy efforts with inspections of prisons and insane asylums throughout Massachusetts and other states and then internationally to England and Scotland (petitioning Queen Victoria for reforms), France and Italy (petitioning Pope Pius IX), and Turkey (trying unsuccessfully to meet with and petition Florence Nightingale at the end of the Crimean War).[25] After Dix's stint as superintendent of women nurses for the Union Army during the US Civil War, she again took up her mental health reform efforts and extended them to the far West, visiting California, Oregon, and Washington Territory. After remarking on the natural beauty of Washington, including snow-capped Mount Rainier, she described in a letter to British Quaker reform friends, the Rathbones of Liverpool, that she was favorably impressed by the Pacific Northwest's "humane and liberal" prisons and insane asylums. She attributed their excellence to how newly settled the area was, a newness that allowed for more progressive thinking than in European or the American East Coast cities.[26]

Dix's trip to the Pacific Northwest was after the time that Edward Moore was living and being cared for by residents of Seattle and Washington Territory. At the time of her visit, Seattle–King County and all of Washington Territory were still using the contract system used with Moore—the auctioning off and contracting out of paupers and people with mental illness. In her report to the Washington territorial legislature, Dix pointed out the abuses of the contract system and recommended that "an experienced medical man" be appointed to supervise the treatment of mentally ill patients.[27]

Dix was involved with political debates raging in England and Scotland, where local parishes used the contract system, paying for their insane poor to live and work in private, for-profit insane asylums. Many of the asylum proprietors cut costs and increased profits by shackling patients in unheated rooms and depriving them of food and medical care. Known as the "trade in lunacy" once the truths were uncovered, the practice was a source of widespread moral outrage and calls for reform.[28] In America, there were claims that the treatment of insane incurable paupers in state-run asylums was a more humane approach. Proponents also said it would save money in the long run, given economies of scale and since patients were not being sent to higher-cost jails and prisons.

Early reports from institutions such as the Worcester Insane Asylum claimed high success rates of "curing" patients of their insanity by citing high patient discharge rates. What they failed to mention were the equally high rates of readmission of these patients to the same or similar institutions within short periods of time. Once forced to face these statistics, proponents of insane asylums, including Dorothea Dix, began to point to "seasonable care," meaning that successful treatment and cure rates occurred when patients were identified early in their illness and were provided with appropriate treatment at insane asylums. "Early" in their illness was typically defined as treatment within the first year of onset of their symptoms.[29]

Public and private debates in America were questioning whether paupers—insane or not—brought on their own plights through immoral acts such as intemperance, specifically in terms of alcohol consumption, and whether it was the duty of the state to care for such people. Calvinist work ethics and conceptions of sin and salvation colored these debates. Women with children born "out of wedlock" and prostitutes were labeled as sinners and as undeserving poor. Leading reformers such as Dorothea Dix declared that the duty of society was the same whether insanity or destitution resulted from "a life of sin or pure misfortune."[30]

There are no indications that Edward Moore exhibited intemperance; if he had been a drinker, that fact would have disqualified him from having legitimate claims to assistance from the residents of Seattle–King County. A curious sidenote about Moore's behavior, as recorded by M. P. Burns, the Steilacoom doctor who took over his care from Maynard, was that Burns found "it necessary to keep said pauper confined hand and foot, in order to keep him from certain habits into which he has fallen and supposed to be the original cause of his present deplorable condition."[31] This was not likely a reference to drinking alcohol as Burns would have stated that fact. It is plausible that Burns's statement about the "cause" of Moore's insanity was a polite and indirect reference to masturbation, as indicated by the shackling of his hands. During that time, masturbation was widely accepted in medical circles as being a direct cause of insanity and even death. Indeed, people were hospitalized and treated for the disease of masturbation, also termed "onanism," and it was viewed as a cause of hereditary insanity.[32]

■ ■ ■

In December 1855, the King County commissioners submitted a report to the Washington territorial legislature requesting reimbursement for the costs of caring for "the lunatic pauper named Edward Moore."[33] The itemized bill for $621 they presented to the legislature included costs for medical attention, nursing, and board for Moore's stay in Seattle. In addition, the bill included costs for Dr. Burns of Steilacoom for medical care, room, and board, the vaguely worded "attendance of a man," and new clothing for Moore; the total bill for Burns was $1,038. The aggregate bill presented to the legislature was $1,659 for the care of Moore over a twelve-month period after he was found on the beach in Seattle.[34]

It is curious but not surprising that the itemized bill presented for the care of Moore did not include costs of the medical and nursing care provided by Doc Maynard and his wife, Catherine. In Seattle, the cost of medical care was linked to a Dr. Williamson, and the cost of nursing care was attributed to David Maurer, the innkeeper. In the legislative report, it was mentioned that Moore was "kept under medical treatment at Seattle, in King County, for four months, partly sustained by voluntary contributions."[35] Doc Maynard was known for his liberal bestowing of free charity medical care, including for Chief Seattle, to the consternation of many of the leaders of Seattle as well as other physicians moving to the area. Catherine Maynard would have followed her husband's wishes in this matter and not billed the territorial legislature for her nursing services for Moore. Maurer charged for nursing services, but he was not a nurse by any stretch of the definition at that time.

In the legislative report, it was noted that Edward Moore was deemed a "nonresident" because of a lack of sufficient evidence that he was a citizen of King County, and it was doubted that "he was ever a resident of Washington Territory."[36] Instead, it established that from what little was known about Moore, he was from Worcester County, Massachusetts, and had a wife and young children living there. No mention was made in this report of any knowledge of other family members. The Poor Laws of Washington Territory stipulated that "every poor person who shall be unable to earn a livelihood in consequence of bodily infirmity, idiocy, lunacy or other cause, shall be supported by the father, grandfather, mother, grandmother, children, grandchildren, brothers or sisters of such poor person, if they or either of them be of sufficient ability."[37] The Poor Laws also authorized counties to charge the relatives of a pauper thirty dollars a month for their upkeep, whether the relatives lived in the county or not.

The legislative committee reviewing the case of Edward Moore decided that although his situation "should touch all the finer feelings of nature," it would be unwise for the legislature "at this early date of our territorial existence . . . to pass a law for the relief of those interested, because it would be setting a precedent that would, if carried out, bring a heavy burden of taxation on the people of the Territory."[38] The total income of Washington Territory from all tax revenue that year was $1,199.88, which was $459 less than the total bill submitted for the care of Moore. The committee also stated that the existing territorial Act Relating to the Support of the Poor was sufficient to "govern in all such cases," and thus it returned the issue to the King County commissioners to deal with. There is no record of the King County commissioners attempting to contact any of Moore's family or the Worcester County, Massachusetts, authorities for reimbursement for the cost of his care. This is not surprising given the slow, cumbersome, and expensive communication channels of the time and the distance between the locations.

In their ruling on this matter, the legislators adopted a preamble and resolution to accompany their decision in the case of Edward Moore. In the preamble, they refer to the issue of the reliance on an increasing number of seamen in Washington Territory in support of the lumber and shipping industries, and the fact that among the sailors "there are many cases of sickness and destitution," creating a burden on the coastal counties like King County and the growing port cities like Seattle.[39] Remembering the by then well-established American practice of conscripting able-bodied male paupers as sailors, this fact is not surprising.

The resolution of the King County commissioners was to have their delegate in the US Congress push for federal funds to erect a marine hospital and an insane asylum in the Puget Sound region. Soon after this, they were successful in procuring federal funds and a site at Port Townsend (less than thirty miles from Seattle by boat) for a marine hospital to take care of "seamen, sick from any cause." Fifteen years later, Congress appropriated funds for the care of the insane in Washington Territory and, later still, land and funding to open the insane asylum at Fort Steilacoom that became Western State Hospital.[40] At the time, the federal government's role in poor relief was largely restricted to welfare aid to war veterans and their widows, although it was being expanded to other "wards" of the nation, including Native Americans and indigent merchant seamen.[41]

■ ■ ■

When Burns of Steilacoom heard of the ruling by the Washington territorial legislature not authorizing reimbursement for his care of Edward Moore, he promptly unshackled Moore, put him in a canoe, paddled him back to Seattle, and left him there. This likely occurred in early January 1856 soon after the legislature's decision, which meant that Moore was living in Seattle during the short-lived but intense Battle of Seattle. In late January 1856, at the height of the fighting between various Indigenous tribes defending their lands and white settlers in the area staking claims to the land, the Seattle townspeople would have bundled Moore into the windowless wood-plank blockhouse for protection from gun and cannon fire—including "friendly fire" from the USS *Decatur* warship situated in Puget Sound near the wharf at Yesler's sawmill.[42] This atmosphere would hardly have been conducive to healing whatever mental illness Moore was suffering from. Afterward, it appears that he was left to fend for himself. He likely wandered around Seattle, lived off whatever handouts and foraged shellfish and berries he could find, and perhaps once again lived in a makeshift tent on the beach where he had been found half frozen and insane the previous winter.

Of note is the mention in various reports that the Native people living on the Seattle beach near where Moore was originally found not only were tolerant of his odd behavior but also helped him survive. This Belltown shoreline had long been an important camping area for Indigenous people, including visitors and migrants from Washington's Pacific Coast, Alaska, and British Columbia. These were not the groups of Native people who attacked Seattle, as they were friendly with the settlers, and many of them worked in the growing fishing and logging industries in and around Seattle.[43]

Considering the situation of Edward Moore and the understanding and treatment of his mental illness in the Seattle area, it is important to point out that Indigenous peoples had much different conceptions of and treatments for what western medicine then termed "insanity" and now terms "mental illness." What western medicine would diagnose currently as depression, mania, anxiety, schizophrenia, or even alcoholism and substance use disorder were considered forms of "spirit illness" and were treated by traditional healers through the use of sweat lodges and spirit dances. Significantly, this treatment involved the person's entire community and not just their immediate family.[44]

The Coast Salish peoples and more inland Indigenous tribes of Washington and Oregon Territories had a Chinook Jargon (the common trading language) word for insanity or "crazy"; that word was *pelton*. This term derived from Archibald Pelton, who was a teenager from New England in an explorer's party following behind Lewis and Clark when they made their way across America to the Pacific Northwest.[45] Pelton's party was attacked by Native people when they reached Oregon Territory. Pelton witnessed the killing of all the men of his party and then was left to wander for months, lost and surviving as best he could on his own until he was found and cared for by another Native tribe. According to various documents from fur traders and settlers who came to know Pelton, it was from this traumatic experience that he became mentally deranged. Pelton was described as having lucid moments during which he could recall some of his experiences, and he became known as an excellent logger. He was killed with his own ax by an Indigenous man who mistook him for another "Boston" (the generic term at the time for American settlers) who had killed the man's friend. The frequent exposure to violence and chaotic frontier vigilante justice, combined with social isolation in the rugged Pacific Northwest, was thought by white settlers of the time to contribute to mental derangement and suicide. The Indigenous people of the Seattle area likely referred to Edward Moore as being pelton and viewed him as harmless and in need of looking after since he apparently had no family to care for him.[46]

There are no indications that Moore was ever shackled or otherwise confined during his time in Seattle as he had been in Steilacoom while under the care of Burns. There are no mentions that he exhibited any violent behavior. Moore was described as "crazy," "odd," and "insane" by various physicians who treated him. But beyond these nebulous terms and the testimony to the Washington territorial legislature by Burns, there are no records of anything Moore said or did while he lived in Washington. Given what is known about Moore—especially considering what became of him—he may have had a form of psychosis, perhaps psychotic depression or, more likely, schizophrenia.

Moore shows up once again in the King County records in the summer of 1856: "The county commissioners decided that Edward Moore, the pauper, now in Seattle, be sold at public auction to the lowest bidder for his maintenance to be paid out of the county treasury, said bid to be left discretionary with the Commissioners to accept or reject, on Saturday, the 7th day of June at 2 o'clock in the town of Seattle."[47] It appears that either no one in Seattle wanted to care for Moore or that the bids were too high and the King County commissioners rejected them. Later that summer, the residents of Seattle–King County collected private donations, bought Moore a new set of clothes, and paid a ship's captain to transport him back to Boston via San Francisco.

All Seattle historians who have included the story of Edward Moore conclude along the lines of Thomas W. Prosch: "What became of him is unknown."[48] I wonder if it was a lack of curiosity, a dismissive attitude toward the significance of Edward Moore as a person, or a lack of modern search capacities for official records that has long had Moore simply disappear in the summer of 1856 onto the ship bound for Boston. But Moore's story does not end there.

■ ■ ■

Fifty miles northwest of Boston, along the watersheds of the Connecticut and Merrimack Rivers in the mill town of Ashburnham in Worcester County, Massachusetts, Edward Moore returned to live with his family members sometime in early 1857. He had survived the six-month treacherous sea voyage around Cape Horn from Seattle to Boston, where he was likely transferred by the ship's captain into the care of his family. Moore had a wife, Rachel, but where she was living at the time and whether she and Moore had any living children together are both unclear. Perhaps Moore tried to visit her once he returned to Massachusetts and was rebuffed due to his poverty and insanity. Rachel Moore probably was living with her parents and perhaps her and Edward's young children in another part of the state.

Whether any of Moore's relatives considered sending him to the Worcester Insane Asylum is unknown. There was no insane asylum in Ashburnham at the time of Moore's return, but there was a town poor farm, which had opened in 1839. Before that, Ashburnham "sold to the lowest bidder" the town's paupers, and the people taking on the care of the poor were called, morbidly, "undertakers."[49] In any case, according to the laws of Massachusetts at the time, the duty to support the "insane pauper" in the Moore family would have fallen to Edward's parents and then his siblings before the town or county stepped in to provide aid.

The forests on the hills around Ashburnham were rich in red oak and chestnut trees, which were milled in town by water-powered machines and turned into furniture, especially chairs, for which the area had become famous by the mid-1800s. Edward's younger sister, Abigail, had married Luke Marble, who owned a lumber and furniture mill in Ashburnham. The Marbles were an old and prominent family in the town. Pitt Moore, Edward's father, then age sixty-nine, and Edward's mother, Esther, age fifty-six, were considered elderly by then and were living with Luke and Abigail Marble, who had three small boys and a daughter on the way. Edward Moore's two older half brothers, Asher and Elliot, were also living in Ashburnham with their wives and young children.[50] Both brothers held town offices. Elliot was a schoolteacher and a town selectman, the assessor, and a member of the school committee. Asher was a farmer and had also been a town selectman. Once he returned to Massachusetts, Edward Moore most likely lived with his parents, sister, and brother-in-law in a wood-framed house near Marble Mill in central Ashburnham, with his half brothers perhaps providing additional financial support for his care.

Edward Moore had been born on January 28, 1823, in Worcester County, Massachusetts, in the rural village of Boylston, less than thirty miles from Ashburnham. Moore died in Ashburnham only a few years after he had been shipped back home by the residents of Seattle. The official notice records his date of death as May 12, 1859, with the cause of death "suicide by hanging (cause insanity)." In the death register, he is listed as being the son of Pitt Moore, married, and without an occupation.[51] Edward Moore is buried beside his parents and other family members in the old cemetery on Meetinghouse Hill in Ashburnham, just north of town on a rise overlooking the Upper Naukeag Lake. His lichen-covered granite gravestone is engraved "Edward Moore / Deceased May 11, 1859 / AE. 36 yrs. 3 ms. 13 ds" (AE is an abbreviation for the Latin *aetatis*, or years of life).

It is intriguing that the date of death on his tombstone and in the official death record differ by one day. Perhaps his family knew that he killed himself on Wednesday, May 11, but his death wasn't certified by a doctor and registered by the town officials until the following day. Exactly where in Ashburnham he hung himself is not recorded. Since it seems he did not exhibit any violent or unruly behavior, and since his family evidently knew that the date of his death differed from the official death date, it is likely that he hung himself at or near the family home where he was living.

When Ezra S. Stearns wrote the lengthy 1887 *History of Ashburnham, Massachusetts*, he included in the chapter "Mortuary Records" a section on suicides.[52] Stearns says, "There was a time when the suicide was denied the rites of Christian burial and his memory was a reproach to his kindred. Perhaps in every instance, certainly in nearly all, the taint of insanity has been manifested in the families in which self-destruction has occurred." He concludes this section by listing the names, ages, and dates of death of the fourteen townsfolk "who have fallen by the cruelty of their own hands." Although the book's time span and location should have included Edward Moore's death from suicide, he is not mentioned in this list. Perhaps Moore was not considered a resident of Ashburnham, or perhaps the Marbles were too prominent a family and the "taint of insanity" so great that they kept his suicide out of this record published by the town.

Would Edward Moore's life have been better—and longer—if he had stayed in Seattle and not been sent back to his family in Massachusetts? Was the initial episode of almost freezing to death on the Seattle beach an early suicide attempt?

These questions, along with many others about the life and death of Edward Moore, Seattle's first homeless person, remain unanswered. We are left with fragments of Moore's life that do not lend themselves to a neat conclusion. Yet his legacy remains. His life in Seattle–King County influenced how the residents and officials have dealt with the quandary of what to do about the increasing number of ill paupers and homeless people, including Native Americans, living—and dying—in their midst.

2

SKID ROAD

Her actions spoke louder than any words she would ever speak.
This was truly her home and she wasn't going to leave.
—Julia Anne Allain, "Duwamish History in Duwamish Voices:
Weaving Our Family Stories since Colonization"

In 1890, along the same stretch of Seattle waterfront where Edward Moore had been found with frozen toes almost four decades before, the piercing cries of seagulls hovering over the city had grown louder. The birds fed off the man-made refuse tumbling down steep hillsides into the tidal flats. On the rise of the hill above this beach, an old woman lived in a six-by-seven-foot one-room windowless home built of cast-off lumber from Henry Yesler's sawmill. Her home was heated by a rusty wood stove.[1] A small dog was her only constant companion. Her deeply furrowed and tanned face was framed by a red bandanna tied under her chin, covering her long black and silver-streaked braided hair. She wore a frayed plaid wool Hudson's Bay blanket across her shoulders that was held closed in front by a large metal safety pin. Under the blanket, layers of old shirts and long, faded calico skirts covered her body—cast-off clothing given to her by white female settlers in partial payment for her work as a laundress. She preferred staying barefoot in all but the coldest weather, walking the beach in search of clams to sell or along the town's growing assortment of dirt streets.

Kikisoblu, known to Seattle townspeople as Angeline, or even Princess Angeline, lived in an area that by 1890 was known as Shantytown.[2] She had lived along this beach for much of her life, and she may have helped Edward Moore survive when he lived there in his makeshift shelter. The daughter of Chief Seattle, Kikisoblu had been a young widow in 1853 when the second wife of settler David "Doc" Maynard, Catherine, met and befriended her. "You are far too handsome a woman to carry that name and I hereby christen you 'Angeline,'" Catherine is reported to have said.[3] That true friends among equals would ever do or say such a thing is unlikely even in that time period in the Pacific Northwest. We do not know what Kikisoblu thought of the presumption of a white woman who renamed an Indigenous woman she had just met, but it seems that Kikisoblu tolerated being called Angeline, or Princess Angeline, at least by Catherine and other early Seattle settlers. It also appears that she considered Doc and Catherine Maynard and the mill owner Henry Yesler to be her friends throughout her long life.

Angeline's home in Shantytown was located along Western Avenue on the downward slope side of Pike Place Market—Seattle's first sanitary market—which began to form in 1896 and officially opened in 1907. Shantytown, photographs of which look eerily like the modern-day Seattle tiny house villages composed of one-room wood structures built on rubble-strewn, city-owned lots, was considered by many people, including city officials, to be an early form of urban blight and a public health hazard. Shantytown had no running water and only a few scattered outhouses. The residents of Shantytown included urban Indigenous people like Kikisoblu, recent immigrants, migrant workers, and families who were too poor to afford other housing options in Seattle—or who were excluded from housing due to their race or ethnicity.[4] Although Seattle and Washington Territory were founded on egalitarian ideals, and the first Washington State Legislature of 1890 passed a public accommodation law specifically prohibiting racial discrimination, such discrimination existed in practice.[5] The residents of Shantytown did not own either their makeshift houses or the land their shacks were built on and were, essentially, squatters.

Unlike the much larger town of San Francisco, California, Seattle's gold was land, and the rush, which was more of a saunter, was by men to claim, settle, develop, and eventually own and sell land in and around Seattle. This was, after all, during the height of the manifest destiny march across the North American continent with the US government's encouragement of settlement across the western frontier.[6] This land rush started with the 1850 Donation Land Claim Act and expanded during the US Civil War with the 1862 Homestead Act. In effect, it was an adaptation and continuance of Britain's practice of welfare colonialism applied to what was then referred to as the New World.

Waves of America's refuse in the form of "poor trash" people—including Irish immigrants fleeing persecution and famine in their homeland—were pushed to the margins of the expanding westward march of what would become the continental United States. Benjamin Franklin, the ultimate proponent of the deep "pull yourself up by your bootstraps" American metaphor of personal transformation through hard work, openly despised poor people and advocated for sending them to the western frontier, which during his time was western Pennsylvania. Franklin viewed this practice as a survival-of-the-fittest sort of endeavor that would simultaneously rid the East Coast cities of urban blight, force the assimilation of immigrants, and improve the character of Americans.[7]

The 1872 painting *American Progress* by Brooklyn artist and lithographer John Gast vividly portrays these concepts. Commissioned by a New York City publisher to accompany a popular series of travel books about the West, *American Progress* is a bird's-eye view of the entire North American continent "from sea to shining sea." On the right-hand side of the painting, there are East Coast cities with bridges and tall buildings that soar toward the sky, illuminated by the rising sun. On the left, the West Coast is largely in the dark, with snow-capped rugged mountains dominating the area near Seattle; the coastline of the town is obscured by thick gray clouds. Bands of Native people and herds of buffalo are fleeing the white settlers headed west in covered wagons along with the white male hunters, explorers, prospectors, and farmers in the foreground. Hovering in the sky and leading the white vanguard is a scantily clad, buxom, blonde young white woman. This embodiment of "American progress"—a sexy sort of white woman missionary-savior—is holding a volume titled *School Book* in one hand and a telegraph wire in the other, representing education, the technology of communication, and connection with the East Coast and European civilization. Railroad tracks and trains originating from the East Coast trail behind her. Except for a few shadowed and faceless bodies inside one of the covered wagons, and several black-clad indistinct Native women huddled on travois platforms being pulled by fleeing horses, the embodiment of American progress is the only female depicted in the painting. And, besides the Native people, it seems there are only white people populating and settling America. The southern states, with their plantations and formerly enslaved African Americans, are conspicuously absent in this painting, as are Chinese migrants in the gold rush and railroad-building parts of the West.

In 1889, Washington Territory finally had sufficient numbers of American settlers and development to become the forty-second state of the United States of America. The results of the 1890 US Census prompted historian Frederick Jackson Turner to proclaim the end of the American western frontier.[8] When the elderly Kikisoblu was living in a shack along the Seattle waterfront, had the American settler development of Seattle followed the formula for "taming" the West as depicted in the painting *American Progress*? Had the Indigenous people in the Seattle area been eliminated, or at least scattered and placed on reservations to clear the way for white settlers? And what major changes had Kikisoblu, Princess Angeline, seen in this city named for her father, this city where she was now a squatter living in a shack on her ancestral land, which she did not own, this city where so many Indigenous people were—and still are—homeless?

■ ■ ■

Seattle was little more than a narrow strip of shoreline crudely cleared of old-growth forest and Kikisoblu was a young widow with two daughters when the Battle of Seattle occurred in January 1856. Viewed from Elliott Bay, the village was bookended by a squat, square, steeple-adorned, white-painted Methodist church on the far northern side and a two-story grand clapboard hotel—Madame Damnable's—on the southern end. In between the church and the hotel was Yesler's wharf, mill, and the mill's growing sawdust pile steadily filling the marshlands near the hotel. A motley collection of fewer than a dozen log cabins stood along the shoreline. Remnants of cedar longhouses and active seasonal encampments of Indigenous people dotted the areas along the beach to the north of the church and the tideland's marshy area below Yesler's mill and Madame Damnable's hotel. Doc Maynard's combination house, general store, and pharmacy stood between Yesler's mill and Madame Damnable's hotel.

Madame Damnable, whose birth name was Mary Ann Boyer, has been described as an illiterate Irish woman.[9] At the age of thirty, with the assistance of Doc Maynard, who provided land along the Seattle shoreline, and financing from Captain Leonard Felker, she built and operated the Felker Hotel, better known as

Madame Damnable's. As an unmarried woman, she could not legally establish a land claim, but she could operate the hotel. It was located in the block between Jackson and King Streets, a half block west of what was then Commercial Street, now First Avenue. The Cowgirls Saloon is located there now—a western-themed establishment where scantily clad female bartenders dance on the bar and a collection of bras hangs from the ceiling.

By all accounts, Mary Ann Boyer was a capable, irascible, shrewd, no-nonsense woman who frequently cursed loudly in at least six different languages. She was Seattle's first business-woman. There is evidence to suggest that before she came to the Pacific Northwest she had been a madam running a brothel in the Fell's Point area of Baltimore, a major East Coast port city.[10] In Seattle, she competed with Henry Yesler and rented rooms in her hotel for nine dollars a night and meeting space for twenty-five dollars to the Washington territorial legislators when they met in Seattle.[11] She reportedly threw sticks of firewood at a leg-islator who asked her for a receipt. It was on the front porch of Madame Damnable's hotel that a "footloose drifter whom no one seemed to know very well—he was variously named in reminis-cences as White, Pocock, and Wilson"—was shot and killed by Indigenous men during the late January 1856 Battle of Seattle.[12]

Running downhill from the forest to Yesler's mill was the de facto dividing line between the town's attempt at piousness and its much more prevalent raucousness. This border, called the dead-line, was Mill Street, known as Skid Road. The dead-line was the result of an early dispute between the founding fathers of Seattle, Doc Maynard, Arthur Denny, and Carson Boren, as to the best layout of the streets. Denny and Boren laid out their streets to run parallel to the shoreline while the scientific May-nard used the points of a compass for his streets. No compro-mise was reached so Yesler Way stands out on maps today as a fault line—and it coincides with the more recently documented Seattle geological fault line for destructive earthquakes.

Skid Road in Seattle, once Mill Street and now Yesler Way, soon became synonymous with people on the down and out—on the skids—people mired in poverty, homelessness or near homelessness, alcoholism, prostitution, and illnesses including tuberculosis, then called consumption for the way the disease consumed or wasted the person's body. Along with the logs that rolled downhill on the skids to Yesler's mill in the early days of Seattle, people figuratively skidded downhill into destitution, illness, and early death. Then, as now, ending up on the skids—or being able to work one's way out of homelessness—was not an equal opportunity affair. Race, gender, sexual orientation, religion, socioeconomic class, exposure to significant trauma, and country of origin all played a role. From Seattle's earliest days, an increasing number of US federal and Washington territorial laws directly benefited Euro-American white men to the detriment of all other people. Most pertinent to the development of Seattle and its perennial homeless problem have been laws pertaining to ownership of housing and land, to marriage and inheritance, and to the treatment of women and of Native American communities. The complexities of these issues can be viewed through the story of Kikisoblu.

■ ■ ■

The eldest daughter of Chief Seattle, Kikisoblu was born sometime around 1820 in the area of South Seattle now called Rainier Beach. Her mother, reportedly a beautiful woman named LaDalia whom Chief Seattle loved, died in childbirth when Kikisoblu was just a few years old. The baby died as well. Kikisoblu was raised alongside her half siblings by Chief Seattle's second wife, Owiyahl. Kikisoblu's childhood nickname was Wee-wy-eke.[13] Her childhood was spent swimming and canoeing and basking in the warmth of being Chief Seattle's daughter.

Arranged marriages between higher-status members of various tribes of the Pacific Northwest were common practice, and in October 1835 Chief Seattle married off Kikisoblu, against her wishes, to Dokubcub, who was of Cowichan and Skagit heritage. Dokubcub paid Chief Seattle ten beaver skins for his new wife.[14] Tellingly, Dokubcub's French Canadian nickname was the Borgne, meaning "one-eyed" or "shifty." The couple moved to Vancouver Island, north of Seattle and now in Canadian British Columbia, where Kikisoblu bore three children, one of whom died soon after birth. Their marriage was tumultuous since Dokubcub was an alcoholic and physically abused Kikisoblu. Duwamish oral histories record stories of Kikisoblu's cunning escape with her two young daughters and her return by canoe to Seattle.[15] Dokubcub was murdered during the winter of 1838, possibly instigated by Chief Seattle in retribution for the ill treatment of his daughter.[16]

Kikisoblu, a young widow raising two daughters on her ancestral land in what became Seattle and its surrounding area, quickly became a well-known and favorite Indigenous woman to the early settlers, or at least to the majority of early settlers. Catherine Maynard not only renamed Kikisoblu, but also taught her how to do the laundry for a growing number of white settler families. Kikisoblu was laundress for the Maynards, including for their small hospital—Seattle's first hospital—which they opened adjacent to their home in 1863. Kikisoblu was the laundress for Madame Damnable's hotel, which was rumored to be Seattle's first unofficial brothel. Kikisoblu also briefly was the laundress for Catharine Blaine, wife of Rev. David Blaine, Seattle's first minister, who built the White Church, the Methodist church with the square steeple north of Skid Road.

Catharine Blaine was an educated young woman from a wealthy family in Seneca Falls, New York, where she had been an eighteen-year-old signatory to the 1848 Seneca Falls Convention's Declaration of Sentiments. She fervently wanted women to gain the vote in order to bring about social reforms, including temperance and women's property rights in marriage. At the time, women lost all property rights when they married.

From her letters written to her parents during her first several years living in Seattle, it is apparent that Catharine Blaine was strongly religious and had married her husband—against her parents' wishes—in a fit of missionary zeal. She had hoped for a missionary post in Africa or China. Instead, she found herself in Seattle where she took an instant dislike to the Indigenous people. She hired and then quickly fired Kikisoblu as a laundress. In a May 3, 1854, letter to her mother, Blaine writes of "turning away" the Native woman, adding, "You talk about the stupidity of the Irish. You ought to work with one of our Indians and then you would know what these words mean."[17] Blaine did her own laundry from then on, pleaded in letters to her parents for special laundry soap to be sent from New York, and became Seattle's first schoolteacher.

Intriguingly, she writes of a shipwreck of the steamer *Southern* in late December 1854. Then, on March 15, 1855, she writes in a letter to her parents of "a crazy man," a "Frenchman, a Physician of very good natural powers, and . . . well educated."[18] Catharine Blaine attributes his mental state to the fact that he lost his wife in France, and he visits their house frequently trying to find a new wife. "I am very much afraid of him," Blaine states. She does not identify him by name, and further references to him do not appear in her surviving letters. Yet she links information on this Frenchman to the plight of another man in Seattle. In the following paragraph, she writes, "Our community, though small, gives an opportunity for the exercise of benevolent feelings. The county has had to take care of a poor, sick, crazy, half frozen man for two or three months past." She indicates that this man, who must have been Edward Moore, "was driven ashore during the strong wind," alluding perhaps to the fact that he had been shipwrecked.

In the aftermath of the Battle of Seattle in January 1856, Catharine Blaine, her husband, and their newborn son fled to Portland, Oregon, where they lived for a while. The Blaines had bought many parcels of Seattle land from which they profited when they returned to live in Seattle in 1882.

During the years that Catharine and David Blaine first lived in Seattle, Kikisoblu's daughter Betsy, who was by then married to a white settler and Washington territorial legislator named Joe Foster, sent word to her mother that she needed help. Betsy had recently given birth to their first—and only—child, a boy named Joe Foster Jr. Joe Foster drank heavily and physically abused Betsy, a fact that seems to have been widely known by the white settlers and the Native people. There were no domestic abuse laws at the time; such abuse was considered a private affair, and wives were considered the property of their husbands. When Kikisoblu arrived at the Seattle beachfront house of the Fosters, she found that her daughter had hung herself in a nearby shed. The date of Betsy's death is recorded by Catharine Blaine as November 22, 1854, which means that Betsy was likely sixteen to seventeen years old when she died.

Catharine Blaine, in a letter to her parents describing this event, tells of her husband refusing to hold a funeral for Betsy when Joe Foster asked him for one. The denial was possibly due to her suicide, but Catharine Blaine states in her letter it was because Rev. Blaine did not recognize them as a "rightfully" married couple since Betsy was Indigenous. She also states that the Native people—including, presumably, Kikisoblu—wanted to have Betsy's body to "bury among their own people, with their own ceremonies," but Foster, "the man who had owned her" refused.[19] Foster had difficulty obtaining a coffin "because she was a squaw" but finally did. Betsy was buried without a Christian service. Catharine Blaine describes her burial: "Indians carried the coffin covered with a blue Indian blanket," and afterward the Indigenous people were "howling and bewailing as they are accustomed to do." She notes that Joe Foster's "half breed child" was "despised by the whites" and that Foster was despised by the Native people for his ill treatment of Betsy. Kikisoblu mourned for her daughter and likely felt deep regret at not being able to prevent either the physical abuse of her by Foster—abuse she herself had suffered in her marriage—or her suicide. After Betsy's death, Kikisoblu raised her grandson Joe Foster Jr. and by all accounts loved and tried to protect him as much as she could. He, in turn, helped her when she became ill in her old age.

■ ■ ■

From its earliest days, Seattle was a rough-and-tumble frontier outpost where Native Americans outnumbered settlers by a large margin and where itinerant single men drifted in and out of the village, mainly working in logging, shipping, fishing, and then the coal mining that developed in the mountains east of Seattle. Historian Coll Thrush estimates that there were a thousand Native people and twenty-four white settlers in Seattle in 1856.[20] Early Seattle also had a severe gender imbalance among the settlers with white men far outnumbering white women.

Many of the male fur trappers and traders with the British Hudson's Bay Company, who had been in the Puget Sound region long before the first American settlers arrived, lived with Native women and were referred to with the offensive term "squaw men."[21] These arrangements were termed "country marriages" for "in the manner of the country."[22] Under the Donation Land Claim Act of 1850, the federal act to establish US claim to what was then Oregon Territory, American men who married Indigenous women were entitled to double the size of their land claim to 640 acres, so many male settlers in the Seattle area took advantage of this until the Washington territorial legislature outlawed such marriages in 1855.[23] It is important to note that unmarried women of any race were not entitled to claim land. This changed later with the Homestead Act of 1862.[24]

Significantly, two of the original founding fathers of Seattle, Henry Yesler and Doc Maynard, had Native American "wives" given to them by Chief Seattle when the men first moved to the area. These unofficial wives were young teenage girls while both Maynard and Yesler were in their forties. Of note, the age of consent for a girl for marriage or sexual intercourse at that time in Washington Territory was twelve.[25] Maynard initially lived with Kikisoblu's daughter Betsy, who was fourteen or fifteen years old. At the time, he was married to his first wife, Lydia, who had stayed behind in Ohio, and he was courting the recently widowed Catherine Troutman Broshears, who was then living with her brother in Olympia south of Seattle. Doc Maynard then conveniently turned out Betsy, marrying her off to another white settler, Joe Foster, before quickly divorcing his first wife and marrying Catherine in January 1853. Indeed, Maynard, in his new role as justice of the peace in Seattle, performed the marriage ceremony between Betsy and Joe.[26] It was this marriage that Rev. Blaine refused to recognize when asked to perform Betsy's funeral just a few years later. Henry Yesler had a daughter, Julia Yesler, with his fifteen-year-old Native American wife, Susan, the daughter of Curley, Chief Seattle's half brother. Julia lived with Yesler even after Yesler's wife from Ohio moved to Seattle in the summer of 1858.[27] Yesler also provided Julia with an education.

It is important to point out the historical context of the complex nature of settler and Native American gendered and racialized relationships. One of the oldest and most enduring stories about this is that of the woman known as Pocahontas, who supposedly saved the life of Captain James Smith, converted to Christianity, and married the Jamestown Colony tobacco farmer John Rolfe. Historian Philip J. Deloria points out that such "romantic race crossing" stories have a long history in America, and they emphasize the access accorded to white men to Native American authenticity and land.[28] The children of these marriages were thought to bring hybrid vigor to the population of the New World, a belief held by Thomas Jefferson.[29] But Indigenous men offering white women access to these same benefits through marriage was, of course, not tolerated due to the gender and social domination patterns that continue in the United States today.

When the first white settlers arrived in Seattle, this race mixing, then known as "amalgamation" or "miscegenation," was frowned upon by the more pious members of the small community. Catharine Blaine, the schoolteacher and minister's wife, referred to men like Doc Maynard, Henry Yesler, and Joe Foster, who all had Native American wives at some point, as debased, godless, and lower-class sorts.[30] Charles Prosch, an early Seattle area newspaperman, writes in his book, *Reminiscences of Washington Territory*, that the practice of white settler men "cohabitating" with Native women "was giving birth to a class of vagabonds who promised to become the most vicious and troublesome element in the population."[31] Prosch points out that the 1855 Washington territorial law against miscegenation could not be enforced "for the reason that too many of the trial jurors as well as the attorneys were in sympathy with the delinquents." Toward the end of his book, Prosch, in his role as a Seattle booster, favorably compares Seattle with East Coast cities. Besides Seattle having a more favorable climate and an abundant food source, "here, beggars, paupers and tramps were unknown; there one could not go out on the public thoroughfares in any direction without encountering the halt, the lame and blind, appealing for a pittance to keep soul and body together."

While Indigenous people outnumbered white settlers in Seattle in its earliest days, African Americans were relatively scarce. The first African American resident, Manuel Lopes, settled in Seattle in 1858 at the age of forty-eight, opening a restaurant and barbershop. A native of Cape Verde off the coast of Africa, islands that were central in the transatlantic slave trade, Lopes moved to New Bedford, Massachusetts, in 1840 as a free man and then worked as a sailor, which is what brought him to Seattle. He lived and worked in the city for at least a dozen years before moving to Port Gamble southwest of Seattle.[32]

Although some white men lived with Indigenous women, there were many white men, especially the loggers and sailors of the region, who were truly single and in search of not only work but also female companionship—and sex—so brothels were established from the very beginning of Seattle. Although Madame Damnable's hotel was rumored to be, at least in its later days, a brothel, Seattle's first official legal brothel was opened in 1861 in the heart of Skid Road by the successful San Francisco brothel owner John Pinnell.[33] He named his Seattle brothel the Illahee, a Chinook Jargon word meaning "home" or "land." The brothel was built on the sawdust-filled area along the waterfront, which was referred to as "down on the sawdust" or the Lava Beds. The prostitutes were all Native American girls and women and were called "sawdust women."[34] In a popular Fraser River, British Columbia, gold rush song, a refrain calls out in fondness the Indigenous prostitutes, clams, and rum at the Seattle Illahee. In addition to brothels, Seattle, as in towns across the West and in Alaska, had a significant number of "cribs," which were small shacks occupied by prostitutes. In Seattle, these blended into the rest of Skid Road alongside other shanties.

It is striking that many male historians refer to prostitution in Seattle as part of the city's culture and the women as just another necessary workforce. Physician James W. Haviland, in his opening chapter of a history of medicine and dentistry in Washington State, describes the early days of Seattle and other Washington towns: "People require services and the necessities of life; and thus we find storekeepers and other traders, prostitutes, bankers, lawyers, and doctors, men and women of the cloth and the churches and the orders they represented all swarming to the newly opened lands."[35] Murray Morgan describes the Seattle waterfront as a place "where you can watch the seamen follow the streetwalkers and the shore patrol follow the sailors."[36] More recently, Coll Thrush states, "Without the labor of Indigenous people—as millworkers and laundresses, clam-diggers and house-builders, prostitutes and potato farmers—Seattle would have been just another failed frontier townsite."[37]

The problem with this view of prostitution is that then, as now, prostitution is not simply sex work on par with being a potato farmer or clam digger, much less a lawyer or doctor. While there may have been an example of a happy, healthy prostitute— Native American or not—in early Seattle, the clear majority of the girls and women who worked as prostitutes came from impoverished, often physical and sexual abuse–filled backgrounds, were of racial and ethnic minority status, and lacked access to education or training for other types of paid work, like being a schoolteacher or nurse. In contrast, most of the men who paid for sex with prostitutes were white, were better educated, and had jobs and money. The prostitutes were exposed to more violence through their work, as well as to diseases like syphilis and tuberculosis. They typically lacked access to healthcare, including safe birth control and abortions, and they suffered from high rates of depression and suicide. They often were lured into prostitution directly from poverty and homelessness and ended up homeless again if they stopped work in the brothels due to age or illness.

Tellingly, the brothels in Seattle's Skid Road red-light district south of Yesler Way were known as "madhouses" for their filth and the frequent screams of women—not in ecstasy but in despair.[38] Even the "high-class" and wealthy Madame Lou Graham, who by the late 1800s was known in Seattle as the Queen of the Lava Beds, died of despondency and suspected suicide in 1903 in San Francisco. She died without a will, and her money went to relatives in Germany and not to the Seattle public schools, although this myth is perpetuated by Bill Speidel in his popular and lucrative tourist attraction, the Seattle Underground Tour.[39]

Madame Graham's four-story brick and stone brothel still stands in the heart of Pioneer Square and is now the Union Gospel Mission's emergency shelter for men.

Throughout the United States and especially in the western territories during the early days of Seattle, there was the common belief that towns and villages needed clearly demarcated red-light districts that included bars and brothels to give men an outlet for their "natural" lust for both alcohol and sex. It was thought that having this separated "vice" section would, in turn, protect "upstanding" girls and women from rape—assuming, of course, that such girls and women knew better than to stray into the red-light district. Seattle's Skid Road, Yesler Way, was the dividing line that served this purpose.

■ ■ ■

Kikisoblu, although she worked as a laundress and housekeeper at Madame Damnable's hotel and perhaps later at official brothels, has never been implicated as having worked as a prostitute. She converted to Catholicism at some point, perhaps in the aftermath of her daughter's suicide, and supported herself and her grandson Joe Foster Jr. by being a laundress and housekeeper, by digging and selling clams, and by making and selling baskets. The Reverend Albert Atwood, a minister who followed Rev. Blaine as the pastor of the White Church, the first church in Seattle, records that "from 1874 to 1877, Angeline resided with queenly grace at the washtub in the parsonage kitchen."[40] He also notes that she was cross with his small children when they got in the way of her work.

In many ways, Kikisoblu as Princess Angeline became a lauded symbol of both the "vanishing race," as depicted in the painting *American Progress*, and the "noble savage." People talked of her as being the "last of her race of people." Stories circulated that she had helped alert settlers to the danger of being attacked before the Battle of Seattle occurred, thus limiting their casualties. She was considered honest, trustworthy, and generous to a fault. Henry Yesler, by then one of Seattle's wealthiest men, when asked why the city was not doing more to support Angeline in her old age, replied that if she was given fifty dollars she would give it all away by nightfall. Of course, she had been raised in an Indigenous culture where wealth is shared, including through the practice of potlatches. Potlatches were important gift exchange ceremonies "in which Natives displayed their wealth, reaffirmed their status, and cemented kinship and community ties."[41] A more modern Tulalip tribal elder from just north of Seattle characterizes potlatches as having the main purpose to "'keep up the poor,' to maintain social cohesion through sharing."[42]

By 1854, there were growing class and racial tensions, especially directed at the continued presence of Indigenous people in Seattle. The Treaty of Point Elliott in 1855, of which Chief Seattle was a signatory, had designated reservations in outlying areas to which the Natives of Puget Sound were supposed to move and become "civilized" by going to "Indian schools," learning to farm, and owning parcels of land. The Duwamish people, of which Seattle was chief, were not given land since white settlers in and around the city claimed it as their own. Many white townspeople falsely equated Native people with contagion, including the dreaded smallpox, and feared they would burn down the mostly wooden structures of the city through their bonfires; the settlers also disliked the shanties and the beach encampments in the city, especially the ones near the Illahee in Skid Road. This culminated with the Seattle Board of Trustees on February 7, 1865, passing Ordinance No. 5, which banned Native people from living in Seattle. An exception was made for those working for Seattle residents like Henry Yesler, in which case the employers were ordered to provide the Indigenous workers with housing on their own property—something they did not do. This law was in effect until the Washington territorial legislature dissolved the government of Seattle in 1867 at the request of the townspeople because of dubious dealings by Seattle officials. Ordinance No. 5 was never reinstated. In any case, Kikisoblu ignored the law and continued to live in Seattle.[43]

Rev. Robert William Summers, the first Episcopal priest of Seattle, wrote about his interactions with Kikisoblu not long after this time. He and his botanist wife, Lucia, were highly educated and avid naturalists. Rev. Summers focused on collecting Native artifacts, known as "curios." Many of the white residents had curio collections in corners of their parlors to show off to visitors. The curios included woven baskets, cedar bark clothing, and even the skulls of Indigenous people.

In January 1871, Rev. Summers writes in his journal of meeting Angeline, who was employed as their laundress. He describes her doing laundry while there was a meeting of the "church ladies" in his parsonage. There was a map of Seattle and the Puget Sound region on the wall near them. Rev. Summers relates that when Angeline saw this map, she became angry. With "eyes aflame and violent stamping," she spoke in Chinook Jargon that her father had *hui illihie* (much land), pointing out lakes, rivers, and villages on the map and stating, "This was his village; this was his home; called by his name Se-at-tle."[44] Rev. Summers also writes of visiting her at her beach home in Seattle soon after this map incident. His visit does not appear to have been on official church business but rather to satisfy his curiosity about Kikisoblu. He describes her dwelling in detail, including that it had "two strong cedar posts" at the front and a door made of a woven mat. Inside, there was a crude fireplace, a bed with a "coarse mat of rushes," a few items of clothing, a wooden bowl, a spoon made of ash, drying racks of fish, and "some very old matting-sacks," sacks that he tried to convince her to part with because he wanted them for his collection. She refused. These sacks were likely used to collect, carry, and sell clams. He writes that she "resent[ed] our visit to such an extent that our investigations [were] rather meagre," and they left. Indeed, one wonders how

Kikisoblu tolerated such an uninvited intrusion into her private space, into her home, at all.

A major fire occurred in Seattle in June 1889 that destroyed much of the downtown area, but it was started accidentally by a young Swedish immigrant man who overturned a glue pot in a furniture store—and not by Indigenous people. At the beginning of the blaze, wood shanties along Yesler Way were ordered destroyed by the mayor in an attempt to stem the spread of the fire. This tactic did not work, and most of the buildings in Skid Road were destroyed. Shantytown on the northern side of downtown, where Kikisoblu lived, was not burned. It is unclear if anyone died in the fire, but city officials later claimed that it had killed a million rats. In the aftermath, housing codes were instituted to require brick and stone buildings, and the previous all-volunteer fire brigade was made into a paid fire department. The city's water supply, which before the fire had been under private control and included the original hollowed-out—and now rotting—fir logs, was replaced, and the city took control of the water supply.

Kikisoblu was strong and capable of protecting herself, and there are many stories of her pelting young boys with rocks and clams when they called her derogatory names in her later years as she walked the streets of Seattle. When US president Benjamin Harrison visited in 1891, Seattle officials arranged for Princess Angeline to sit near him in the newly opened Pioneer Place (now Pioneer Square) rising from the ashes of the fire.[45] She greeted him in Chinook Jargon. After this, city boosters proposed sending Kikisoblu on an around-the-world trip with the eccentric and wealthy land speculator and railroad tycoon George Francis Train, who had been the inspiration for the popular book by Jules Verne, *Around the World in Eighty Days* (1872). Angeline told a newspaperman that she "wanted no truck" with Train.[46]

Photographers began to seek out Kikisoblu as a subject, and in turn she began to charge one dollar as a sitting fee. The now-famous photographer Edward S. Curtis took pictures of Kikisoblu both in his studio and likely on the Seattle beach as she dug for clams. These photographs with Angeline as the subject launched his career as a photographer of the "vanishing race" of Native Americans across the American West. Many other less-famous photographers also took pictures of "Princess" or even "Queen" Angeline. These photographs, often heavily edited, made their way onto thousands of postcards that were sold in stores in Seattle and throughout the Pacific Northwest. Except for the occasional sitting fees she managed to charge for photographs, Kikisoblu did not profit from the sales of her likeness.

After she was found to have a poorly mended broken wrist from a fall, Kikisoblu became a ward of King County. A shopkeeper near her shack was instructed to give her an open line of credit. She stomped her wood cane on the floor of the shop when she felt she was being given an inferior cut of meat. Her monthly grocery bill never exceeded three dollars.[47] The Reverend R. W. Summers in his *Indian Journal* writes in 1890 of Chief Seattle and Kikisoblu, "The city should kindly care for his daughter, poor old Angeline Seattle, who at the time of this writing is a beggar in the streets of uplifting commercial palaces and lovely homes!"[48] Where he got the idea that she was a beggar is not known, unless he is referring to her being a county ward. The only other description of Angeline ever begging for anything is by Bertha Piper Venen in her overwrought book of verse, *Annals of Old Angeline*, where she indicates that Angeline sometimes asked for a cigarette from men smoking on the streets.[49]

The Duwamish were never given the land promised to them in the treaties, and today they remain unrecognized as a tribe by the federal government. It is known that Kikisoblu deeply resented the loss of all her father's land, as vividly recounted by Rev. Summers. An oft-repeated anecdote is that she ran up to one of the founders of Seattle, Arthur Denny, when she saw him on the street and exclaimed, "God damn you! Mr. Denny.

God damn you!" Denny laughed and thought she meant to say, "God bless you!" It is more likely that she knew exactly what she was saying.

Kikisoblu's second daughter, Mary, had married a white man, William DeShaw, who ran the Bonanza Trading Post on Bainbridge Island near Seattle. His trading post was near Old Man's House on Agate Pass, the traditional winter home of Chief Seattle and his Suquamish relatives. After Chief Seattle's death in 1866, William DeShaw was appointed Indian agent and was instructed to move the Indigenous people from the large, communal (and communist in the eyes of many white people) living area of Old Man's House to the nearby reservation and to force them to live in individual homes. DeShaw burned down what remained of Old Man's House although many of the Native people continued to camp among its remains.[50]

As she grew older, Kikisoblu often sat to rest in store doorways or on the curbs of the raised wooden sidewalks in downtown Seattle. The Archdiocese of Seattle records that she was often seen on the streets with a cigarette in her mouth and a rosary in her hands.[51] Later, townspeople found her fallen on the street and unable to walk. They tried to take her to the nearby Seattle General Hospital, but she refused and called it a jail and a "house of ghosts"—she viewed the hospital simply as a place where people went to die. She returned home to her shanty under the care of her grandson Joe Foster Jr. She refused medications from the white physician who visited her and who diagnosed her with consumption (tuberculosis). By then, Doc Maynard, the one physician she had trusted, was dead. Kikisoblu asked Joe to fetch traditional herbs for a tea to help her regain her strength.

Seattle officials decided to build her a new house adjacent to her old one, which they then tore down. In photos, this new house is only marginally better than the first one. Soon after the move, she died in her home in Shantytown on May 31, 1896.[52] According to her wishes, as they were relayed to Catherine Maynard, who outlived her, Angeline was buried in a coffin shaped like a canoe and was interred next to her friend Henry Yesler. She wore her red bandanna and a brown shroud.[53] Her grandson Joe Foster Jr. was the only Native person to attend her funeral service in the Catholic church. He had developed a drinking problem and continued to live in Angeline's shack until the land it was on was cleared to make way for Pike Place Market. What became of him is unknown. Besides Princess Angeline's gravestone in Lake View Cemetery in Seattle, the only other marker of her existence is the YWCA women's shelter in Belltown near where she lived in Shantytown. It is named Angeline's Day Center for Women and is a safe house for women dealing with intimate partner violence, prostitution, and homelessness.

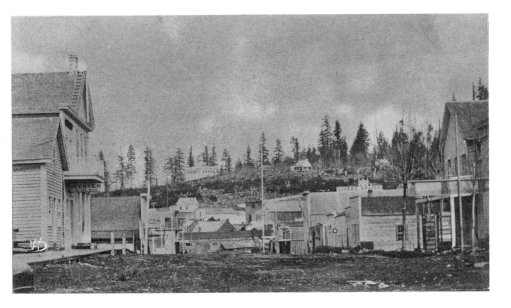

Commercial Street looking north, Seattle, 1865.

Far left, Seattle Hospital; *center on hill in background*, the university;

far right, Doc Maynard's home.

Source: Museum of History and Industry, Seattle, MOHAI, shs239.

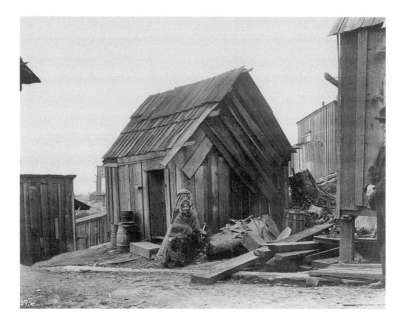

Princess Angeline seated in front of her wooden house.

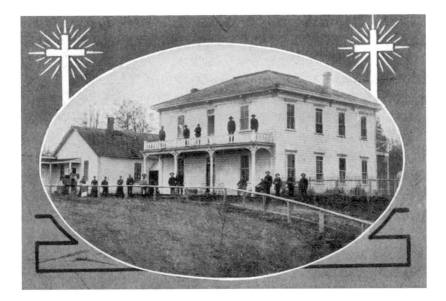

King County Poor Farm in Georgetown, 1870s.

Source: Providence Archives, Seattle, 56.A1.2.

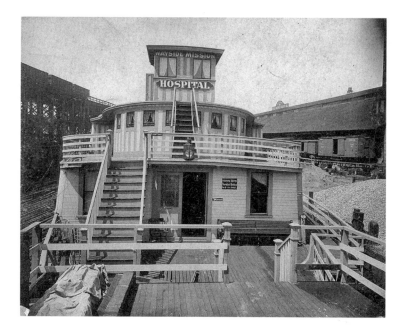

Entrance to the Wayside Mission Hospital housed
on the steamboat *Idaho*, Seattle, circa 1900.

Source: University of Washington Libraries, Special
Collections, Seattle, UW 6573.

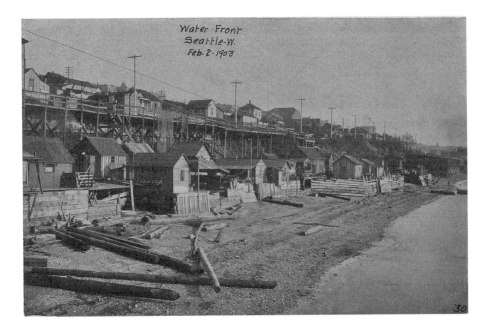

Beach shacks on the waterfront, Seattle, 1903.

Source: Museum of History and Industry, Seattle, MOHAI,

Benjamin Pettit Photograph Collection, 1980.6923.108.

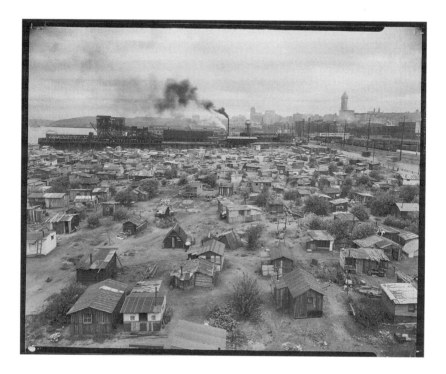

Hooverville, Seattle, March 1933.

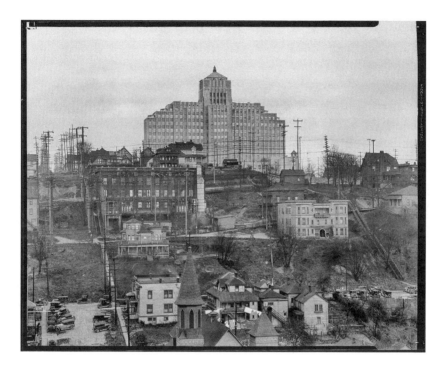

Harborview Hospital, Seattle, 1931.

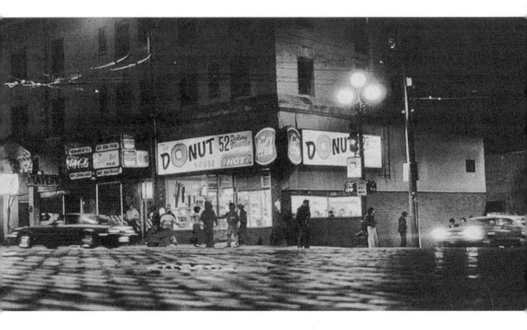

The Donut House, 1981.

Source: Museum of History and Industry, Seattle, MOHAI,
Seattle Post-Intelligencer Collection, 2000.107.172.01.02.

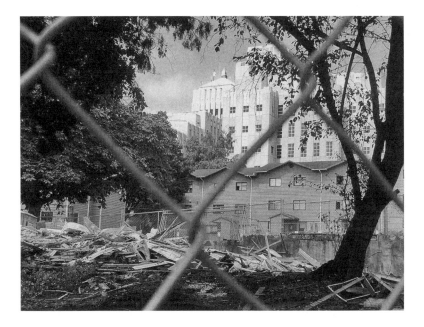

Demolition of Yesler Terrace with Harborview
Medical Center in background, 2015.

Source: Photo by author.

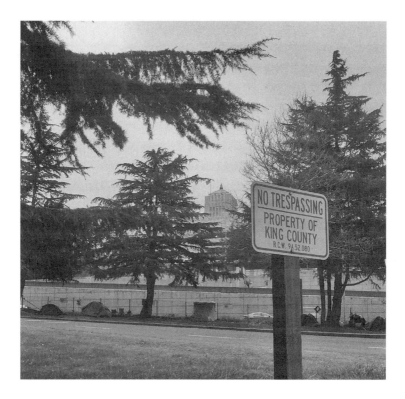

Tent encampment, Yesler Way, Seattle, 2015.

Source: Photo by author.

3

THE SISTERS

Charity is one of those remarkable words that helps
to identify the fault lines of a culture.

—Janet Poppendieck, *Sweet Charity? Emergency Food
and the End of Entitlement*

Late on the evening of May 3, 1877, three women dressed head
to toe in heavy, black wool clothing stepped off the side-wheeler
steamboat *Alida* from Fort Vancouver in Washington Territory
onto the boat landing at the end of Mill Street in Seattle. Sister Blandina of the Angels, Sister Peter Claver, and Sister Mary
Aegedius, all from the Catholic order Sisters of Charity of Providence, had arrived to assume responsibility for the running of
the King County Poor Farm and Hospital. Originally from Montreal, Canada, their primary language was French, and they were
only haltingly conversant in English.

The Sisters spent their first week in Seattle living with a
Catholic family, preparing linens, and obtaining hospital supplies. Then, on the sunny morning of May 11, they made their
way by horse-drawn carriage on a deeply rutted dirt road—later
to become State Route 99, also known as the Pacific Highway—

four miles south of Seattle to the newly opened Poor Farm and Hospital along the banks of the Duwamish River. All three were nurses, and Sister Peter Claver was trained as a pharmacist. Sister Blandina was the superior of this Seattle mission, and Sister Peter Claver was her assistant. Following the dictates of their faith, the three women eschewed individuality and thus were most often referred to collectively as "the Sisters."[1]

When the Sisters arrived at the foot of Skid Road, King County had a population of just over 5,600 people, with 3,000 residents living in the growing town of Seattle.[2] The year 1876 had seen large growth in the local economy with the completion of the regional railroad between Seattle and the coal mines in Newcastle in the southeastern part of King County. The hop-growing industry was beginning in the fertile river deltas in south King County, including the area of the poor farm. During the following decade, the Seattle area would become the world's largest producer of hops for beer production. More than a hundred new houses had been built in and around the town, new roads and streets were completed, and older streets like Front Street were regraded. Kikisoblu was living in her one-room house in Shantytown. Catherine Maynard had opened a free reading room—the town's first public library—in her house in Pioneer Square.[3]

The most visible building in town was the grand, pillared, and bell-towered Territorial University of Washington. Built on a Seattle hill in 1856, it had just graduated its first university student, Clara Antoinette McCarty, who became a schoolteacher. The university had only sporadically been open since its beginning because it frequently ran out of funding—and students—in the small frontier town. It was closed again for lack of funds when the Sisters arrived. In 1877, Seattle's wealthiest businessman, Henry Yesler, refused to pay the city of Seattle the assessed $5,000 against his sawmill and other properties downtown for the regrading of Front Street. The Pinnell madhouse brothel, the Illahee, had just been closed and would soon mysteriously burn down, to the relief of many residents of Seattle, including the recently arrived Sisters. But numerous brothels and taverns continued to thrive in the area south of Mill Street in the Skid Road part of town.[4]

With the population growth in the Seattle area came an increase in the number of poor, ill, and homeless people, many of whom stayed long enough to become wards of King County. The King County commissioners dealt with such cases one by one: deciding on payment amounts for medical treatment, room, board, and nursing care for such individuals. Essentially, they continued the same contract process that they had applied to the case of Edward Moore, the county's first insane pauper, back in the winter of 1854.

In their official proceedings, the commissioners recorded the names of county paupers along with the decisions about payments to be made to various physicians and other citizens submitting bills for care of the county wards. On December 22, 1866, for example, the commissioners ordered that notices for taking care of the "pauper Shram" be posted, and they authorized the county auditor to accept the lowest bidder to care for him, "the bidder to furnish medicines and all things necessary."[5] In November 1867 David "Doc" Maynard presented a bill of $478.50 to the county commissioners for his care of "Crew, a pauper," but the commissioners only allowed $236 to be paid to Maynard.[6] Henry Yesler was reimbursed for the cost of shipping a pauper back to the Sandwich Islands (Hawaii).[7] In 1873, the King County commissioners tired of their role of hearing and deciding on each pauper, so they appointed an overseer of the poor to perform these duties. The first overseer was Seattle physician T. T. Minor.

The combination of an increase in population and the fact that Seattle was becoming a major port city in the Pacific Northwest led to outbreaks of infectious diseases that were of growing concern to residents and elected officials. Seattle boosters wanted to portray the city as a healthy place for more people to move to—

or, at least, certain types of people. They wanted to attract people who could be upstanding citizens, improve the local economy, and increase the wealth of early landholders. Infectious disease outbreaks were a blight that they wanted eradicated. It did not help that Seattle lacked any real hygiene, water, sanitation services, fire safety, or building standards. Outdoor privies in backyards drained downhill directly into Puget Sound and, often, into wells that supplied drinking water to the population. Rats, first introduced to the area from early European explorers' ships, thrived in the relatively mild climate and in the town full of refuse. The medical and public health understanding of infectious disease etiology, prevention, and treatment remained rudimentary. The germ theory of disease was in its infancy. Outbreaks of communicable diseases like malaria, cholera, typhoid, tuberculosis, measles, and diphtheria regularly affected the population of Seattle. But it was smallpox, which was so highly contagious, deadly, and permanently disfiguring, that was most feared.

Smallpox and malaria were both unknown diseases to Native Americans, who lacked any immunity to them.[8] This susceptibility is thought to be largely responsible for the high mortality rates documented among Indigenous tribes, including those in the Pacific Northwest, upon contact with European colonizers. Ironically, Native Americans were often blamed for disease outbreaks among settlers, especially smallpox. The oldest surviving piece of printed material from Seattle is a handbill titled "Smallpox! City Ordinance No. 30" from July 2, 1872, which was signed by the mayor, who was also Seattle's first health officer, Dr. Gideon A. Weed.[9]

By this time, there was a relatively safe and effective smallpox vaccine, but the main medical and governmental policy approach was early identification of diseased individuals and quarantine of them in their homes, on the ships upon which they had arrived, or in a designated "pest house" established and maintained by the city on the outskirts of town. The city ordinance established mandatory reporting of smallpox patients by physicians, hotel owners, and ship captains; failure to do so could result in police action and fines of between $50 and $500. In addition, it authorized the Seattle health officer to vaccinate people and bill the city. In the winter of 1876–1877, as the three members of the Sisters of Charity of Providence were making plans to move to Seattle, a smallpox epidemic struck the city. Seattle's mayor was still the physician Weed. He began to vaccinate Seattle residents and isolated those who showed symptoms. Despite these efforts, eight people died, five of whom were Native American, so many Seattle residents continued to blame Indigenous people for the scourge. They also equated diseases, such as smallpox and syphilis, with the brothels, saloons, bawdy houses, and shanties of Skid Road.[10]

In addition to the danger of infectious disease outbreaks in the port city, the logging, milling, mining, railroad-building, farming, and fishing industries in and around Seattle had high rates of injuries and illnesses among their workers, who often were single men without families to care for them. Various physicians, including Doc Maynard, provided medical care and primitive surgery for many of the injured and ill people in town, including paupers. Catherine Maynard assisted her husband and provided nursing and midwifery services. They maintained a pharmacy, selling both patent tonics and their own, including dandelion tonic, likely in the form of dandelion wine. Catherine Maynard is credited with cultivating the first dandelions in the Seattle area specifically for medicinal use, including as a treatment for scurvy, which still affected sailors as well as miners in Alaska.[11]

In early December 1863, the Maynards advertised in a Seattle newspaper, the *Gazette*, the opening of their hospital and maternity department.[12] The simply named Seattle Hospital was located on the northwest corner of Commercial (now First) Avenue and Jackson Street, directly across the street from their home, consulting office, and pharmacy. The lying-in (maternity) department was advertised as being "entirely under the care of Mrs. C. T. Maynard." Seattle Hospital, although modest in size, was Seattle and King County's first official hospital, and Catherine Maynard was Seattle and King County's first official nurse. Gideon A. Weed took over the running of Seattle Hospital once Doc Maynard became too ill to continue his medical practice. Maynard died in 1873 at age sixty-four of liver failure, likely the result of decades of heavy drinking.[13]

While the King County commissioners were paying for the medical and social support care for an increasing number of ill paupers, they came into possession of farmland. Through a court case of a man who died without relatives or a will, the county now owned a 160-acre tract of farmland on the Duwamish River south of town in an area known as Georgetown. The commissioners leased the farm to brothel owner John Pinnell—who supervised farming there, mostly of potatoes—and they maintained a county cemetery for paupers on part of the land.

The commissioners decided to open a poor farm and hospital in hopes of containing the rising cost of care for paupers, especially sick or injured paupers who required nursing and medical care. They advertised for bids for medical care, for building the county poorhouse, and for the nursing care of public wards of King County. Father and son physicians A. and H. B. Bagley were awarded $300 for one year for medical and surgical care and provision of medicines to the county poor. Walter Harmon and George Walker were paid $1,400 for completion of the building of the poorhouse by May 15, 1877.[14] This left the nursing care. Although Catherine Maynard was a nurse and there likely were a few other nurses in Seattle by that time, none were prepared to take on the nursing care and administration of the new county hospital. Maynard was now an elderly widow who lived part time with relatives in eastern Washington. Several farmers put in bids to provide nursing care, which they knew nothing about. The King County commissioners turned to Father Modeste Demers, the area's first Catholic priest, who volunteered the Sisters of Charity of Providence to take on the nursing care of ill paupers at the King County Poor Farm and Hospital. Father Demers agreed to lease the county farm for $300 a year and to provide care for the county poor at seventy-five cents per patient per day.[15]

■ ■ ■

Beginning in 1856, the Sisters of Charity of Providence had established hospitals in Portland, Oregon Territory, and in Vancouver, Washington Territory, across the Columbia River from Portland. They viewed their nursing care as an extension of their missionary work in the "land of the infidels." Significantly, they included Protestants in their list of infidels.[16] This was before there were any nursing schools in either Canada or America. The effects of Florence Nightingale's work were just beginning to spread from England. The Sisters' nursing skills were learned by apprenticeship from other nurses in various rudimentary hospitals for the poor and insane in Montreal.

Mother Joseph of the Sacred Heart was their leader in the Pacific Northwest. From her childhood as Esther Pariseau in the Montreal area, she had dreamed of being a missionary on the western frontier. Mother Joseph was a woman of action who loved designing and overseeing the building of hospitals and schools. She was a shrewd and forthright businesswoman. When the Sisters of Charity of Providence ran short of funds for their work, Mother Joseph set off in her black habit on horseback with Native American guides on "begging tours" throughout the state of Oregon and Washington Territory, going to the source of money: the logging and gold-mining camps. She was fond of the beautiful and intelligent young women who came to work with her.[17] She hated housework. In response to a rebuking comment from a priest, she admitted to being aligned more with action than with passive prayer and trust in providence.[18]

Not long after King County cared for Edward Moore and the

county commissioners had appealed to the Washington territorial legislature for assistance with the cost of his care, the legislature contracted with the Sisters of Charity of Providence in Vancouver to care for the territory's growing number of mentally ill poor patients. At the time, families that could afford the cost sent their mentally ill family members to the much larger city of San Francisco for treatment. But Washington Territory had an increasing number of poor and family-less mentally ill people. Territorial legislators were concerned with maintaining the image of Washington Territory as a healthy place for people to move to, and having insane paupers at large in communities did not help this image.

In 1861, Washington Territory paid the Sisters eight dollars a week per patient, and they cared for seventeen mentally ill patients the first year.[19] Their facility in Vancouver was called St. John of God Lunatic Hospital, and it was modeled after the psychiatric facility St. Jean de Dieu Asylum run by their mother house in Montreal. Neither facility was based on the newer moral treatment models of psychiatric care, but the Sisters did maintain cleanliness in the facilities and treated their patients with compassion. By 1866, they had twenty-five mentally ill patients.[20]

The Sisters of Charity of Providence provided care to the territory's mentally ill patients until the end of 1866 when their contract expired. Mother Joseph wanted to extend their contract, but she became mired in a dispute with the territorial legislature over payment. She had requested payment in gold coin, but the legislature had paid her in greenbacks, which had been devalued severely during the Civil War. Mother Joseph figured out the depreciation, plus interest, and demanded $4,000 in payment. She enlisted the help of a lawyer to essentially—and, years later, successfully—sue the territorial legislature for the funds.[21] Her insistence on full payment likely angered some of the legislators, all of whom were men who likely held the prevalent paternalistic views on women's "proper" roles in politics and society. Regardless, the Sisters of Charity of Providence were underbid by two businessmen of Monticello (now Longview), a location much closer to the Washington territorial capital of Olympia. The two men quickly built a rough barn-like structure with individual "cells," and eleven patients were transferred from Vancouver to their new facility in the summer of 1866.[22]

The two businessmen had no experience in the provision of care for mentally ill patients, and they quickly ran into difficulties, with an unmarried female patient becoming pregnant and giving birth while in their facility, and other patients wandering off before they were examined and officially discharged by a physician.[23] In the summer of 1869, during mental health reformer Dorothea Dix's visit to the Pacific Northwest, she reported on the level of filth at the Monticello facility and the fact that many patients were locked in their eight-by-five-foot cells. She recommended to the Washington territorial legislature that the facility be closed and patients sent to the much better, privately run Oregon Insane Hospital in Portland, which she had personally inspected.[24] Oregon had become a state in 1859 while Washington would remain a frontier territory until 1889. In her letter to the legislature, Dix pointed out that Washington was too sparsely populated to support a well-run psychiatric facility, and she highlighted the well-known abuses of the contract system for care of mentally ill patients. The legislators did not heed her advice on this point. They did, however, follow her advice to at least appoint a physician to supervise more closely the care of mentally ill people at their contracted facility.

Dorothea Dix had lobbied persistently in Washington, DC, for the federal government to set aside a portion of its considerable, growing ownership of land for the provision of adequate insane asylums in every state and territory. The Land-Grant Bill for Indigent Insane Persons, dubbed the "ten-million-acre bill," was legislation that Dix helped craft and steer to approval by both the House and Senate in 1854. It was vetoed by the alcoholic and anti-abolitionist President Franklin Pierce, who stated he did not want to make "the Federal Government into the great almoner of public charity throughout the United States."[25] This happened amid raging debates nationally not only about slavery, but also about social welfare and which level of government should pay for and supervise care of the insane, paupers, and homeless people. In the years leading up to the Civil War, the southern states successfully advocated for a weaker federal government and stronger states' rights, including their right to determine how they would care for poor, homeless, and insane people. The federal role in national social welfare continued to be limited to veterans and marines and would not be expanded until the 1930s with the crisis of the Great Depression.[26]

Besides the tenacity of Mother Joseph in demanding payment with interest for the care of insane paupers, an additional reason the Washington territorial legislature transferred the care of mentally ill patients from the Sisters to nonsectarian caregivers was likely related to the separation of church and state. America was founded on the principle of religious freedom, as well as an early awareness of the need for the separation of church and state. Washington Territory included this separation in its territorial constitution, as did King County, and documents for both levels of government also emphasized religious freedom and tolerance.

■ ■ ■

Catholicism has the oldest roots of any organized religion in the Pacific Northwest, as its missionaries had ties with the Montreal-based Northwest Company, which merged with the British Hudson's Bay Company. The Catholics in the Pacific Northwest focused their work among the male French Catholic voyageurs and fur trappers and on converting the Native people, as they did eventually with both Chief Seattle and his daughter Kiki-soblu.[27] The early Catholics in the Pacific Northwest backed the British and not American claims to the land that became the states of Washington and Oregon.[28] One month after Henry Yesler opened his mill in Seattle, Father Demers, the first Catholic bishop of British Columbia, stepped out of a canoe onto the Seattle beach and asked if there were any Catholics for him to minister to. The townspeople answered no but offered to gather people to hear him speak. He spent the night with the staunch Protestant Arthur Denny and his family and the next morning gave a sermon in Yesler's cookhouse. The theme of his sermon was charity, and he repeated the refrain, "Charity, my friends, charity—always charity."[29] While it is unclear to whom those listening that morning should be charitable, it is likely that Father Demers was referring to Native people, new settlers and visitors to the small village, and possibly any paupers who would end up on their shores. In the Catholic faith, charity is defined as the love of God and the love of neighbors as oneself. Along with faith and hope, charity is one of the three main Catholic theological virtues.[30]

Seattle, from its very beginning, was largely developed by people who were tolerant of but mostly indifferent to organized religion. Henry Yesler and his first wife, Sarah, were Spiritualists who believed in having an open marriage. Sarah had at least one passionate relationship with a woman once she moved to Seattle. And Henry had lived with and had a daughter with Chief Seattle's young niece Susan while married to Sarah. Doc Maynard was far from being a believer, a teetotaler, or a churchgoing man. Catherine Maynard had ties to the Christian Church (Disciples of Christ Church), which had roots in Kentucky, where she was raised. In early 1856, when Seattle's first minister, Rev. David Blaine, and his wife, Catherine, fled after the Battle of Seattle, they had four members of their then two-year-old church—and they included themselves in that count.[31] Seattle remains one of the country's most secular cities.[32]

During this time throughout the United States and its territories, Protestantism was viewed by many people as being solidly American, given the country's Puritan roots. Catholicism was viewed as un-American because it was associated with the increasing number of impoverished Irish immigrants and with non-English-speaking immigrants from France, Spain, and Mexico. In the Pacific Northwest, people remembered that the Catholic Church had sided with Britain over the contested land. They also remembered the close ties of Britain with slave-owning southern states during the Civil War. Indeed, in the dispute between Mother Joseph and the Washington territorial legislature over payment, legislators pointed out to her that the Catholic Church had sided with Britain and the US Democratic Party, and therefore they were partially responsible for the devaluation of greenbacks. They also admonished the Sisters to live up to their name and practice charity.[33]

■ ■ ■

The three Sisters—Sister Blandina of the Angels, Sister Peter Claver, and Sister Mary Aegedius—moved to the newly built King County Poor Farm and Hospital on May 15, 1877, and quickly set up the space to suit their needs. Building plans show a two-story wood-frame building fifty by sixty feet with six rooms on each floor. The structure included the Sisters' dormitory, a kitchen, a small chapel, and a parlor on the first floor. The second floor was designated "room for the poor" and could accommodate up to ten patients. The hospital at the poor farm had an outdoor privy and a detached barn and shed for the horses, carriage, and farm equipment. In their *Chronicles*, the Sisters note that it was generally referred to by people in the area as either the "poorhouse" or the "workhouse" and not as a hospital.[34]

The Sisters of Charity of Providence were, for the most part, educated and literate women. During a time when medical records were nonexistent, they kept neat and meticulous patient ledgers. The ledgers included the patient's name; nationality; location of last residence; age; admission, discharge, or death dates; and religion, with a running tally of Catholics versus Protestants. They did not record patient diagnoses in the ledgers until May 1886. They had an official Sister chronicler assigned the duty of recording a detailed account of their spiritual and hospital work—and occasionally the stories of their patients. The *Chronicles* for their early years working in Seattle were written in French and were not signed, so we do not know which Sister kept these journals. They were handwritten in large, leather-bound ledgers. The Sisters made two copies of the original *Chronicles*, with one copy sent to the mother house in Montreal and the other copy sent to Mother Joseph in Vancouver, Washington Territory. The original *Chronicles* were kept at their office in the hospital in King County.[35]

While the *Chronicles* were meant to emphasize the spiritual work of the Sisters, they also documented aspects of their daily lives. In addition, through the *Chronicles*, the Sisters shared their views on local politics and what they saw as ongoing religious bigotry and persecution for their Catholic faith. The *Chronicles* of the Sisters of Charity of Providence make frequent references to their efforts to convert patients to Catholicism, including many deathbed conversions. They describe covert baptisms of infants and small children, including an infant born to a Protestant woman. The mother was adamant that she did not want her child baptized. The Sisters record how they distracted the mother so that another Sister could pour holy water over the child's head before it died.[36]

The Sisters of Charity of Providence admitted their first patient, John Benson, on May 19, 1877. He was a forty-three-year-old white Protestant laborer originally from Norway and living in south King County along the White River, close to the poorhouse. They do not record what his illness or injury was, but they do note that he died at their hospital on July 12 of that same year. Their second patient, Alexander Barrett, a thirty-five-year-old white Catholic laborer living in Seattle but originally from Canada, was admitted on May 24 and died in their hospital on October 28. Their third patient, Mary Tucker, a nineteen-year-old woman from Seattle, was admitted on May 26 and discharged on June 16. She is listed as being Protestant; for country of origin the Sisters wrote "mulatto," a commonly used term then for a person of mixed race, typically a person with one white and one Black parent. No profession is noted for her. Her two-month-old son, John Tucker, was patient number four. He is listed as being "mulatto" and Protestant and was admitted and discharged on the same dates as his mother.[37] Mary Tucker would return to the hospital a few years later under curious circumstances that would affect the work of the Sisters of Charity of Providence in King County.

Some of the patients who were well enough to work helped the Sisters in the hospital, in the kitchen, and on the farm. The farm had a mature orchard of fruit trees and highly productive riverside soil to grow potatoes and other vegetables to augment their food supply, as well as surplus to sell. The land had been the site of an extensive Duwamish fishing village, and the black alluvial soil was enriched by decomposed clam and oyster shells.[38] But most of their patients came to them too ill, injured, old, or infirm to be able to do any work. In their first year of operation of the King County Poor Farm and Hospital, the Sisters cared for thirty patients, ten of whom died during their hospital stay.

The high mortality rate gave the poor farm a reputation of being a house of death, and the Sisters were rumored to be angels of death, ushering people into early deaths and profiting from deathbed conversions, with patients bequeathing them whatever money or valuables they may have had. It did not help that the Sisters wore black habits and were frequently observed talking in French, a language most of their patients and visitors could not understand. Their reputation as angels of death was reinforced by the King County cemetery, Potter's Field, filling with deceased paupers, a cemetery that was in close proximity to the hospital. The Sisters blamed both their low patient census—often fewer than ten patients—and their reputation as a death house on religious bigotry by townsfolk toward their Catholic faith. In their *Chronicles*, the Sisters frequently complain about the distance of the King County Poor Farm and Hospital from the bustling center of Seattle and the designation "poorhouse" as additional reasons for their low patient census.[39]

■ ■ ■

The poorhouse concept was purposefully designed to be a place to be feared, to be a deterrent to idle pauperism, to be a place of last resort even for the worthy poor, including the aged and orphans. Increasingly, unmarried women and their children were considered unworthy poor in both England and America. Like the Elizabethan Poor Laws, the poorhouse or almshouse model was first developed in England and quickly spread to America, first in East Coast cities such as Boston, Philadelphia, and New York.[40] The poor farm model was adopted for more rural towns and agricultural areas of the US states and territories. They all were designed to include paupers' cemeteries as a reminder to poor people that this was their ultimate fate, unless their cadavers were sold to anatomists for use in dissection, ostensibly in the name of science.

By the nineteenth century, the Elizabethan Poor Laws in England, as well as the adaptations of them in America, were under increasing scrutiny, and critics called for radical changes. In England and Scotland, the effects of the land clearances, the enclosures, the rise of the Industrial Revolution, and the Napoleonic Wars created a marked increase in poverty and destitution, especially in urban areas, such as London and Edinburgh. In England, one of the most influential critics of the Poor Laws was the economist and Church of England cleric Robert Malthus. Rev. Malthus contended that public and even Christian charity led to the breeding of yet more paupers. In particular, he placed blame for the rising levels of poverty on unmarried mothers, including prostitutes, and not on the men who fathered the children. Other critics carried this belief further to cast blame on all charitable institutions providing maternity care for poor women and even on orphanages for foundlings.[41]

Jeremy Bentham, the English social reformer, philosopher, and outspoken atheist best known for development of the moral principle of utilitarianism, or the greatest good for the greatest number, influenced subsequent policy changes to the Poor Laws. Bentham developed the model of the panopticon with its central observation platform for prisons, insane asylums, and even hospitals. He believed that the surveillance highlighted by the building design created sufficient anxiety among prisoners and patients to keep them under control by fewer staff, thereby reducing costs. As Michel Foucault states in *Discipline and Punish: The Birth of the Prison*, "The panopticon functions as a kind of laboratory of power. . . . it serves to reform prisoners, but also to treat patients, to instruct schoolchildren, to confine the insane, to supervise workers, to put beggars and idlers to work."[42]

One of Bentham's students, Edwin Chadwick, became the leader of Parliament's Royal Poor Law Commission for Inquiring into the Administration and Practical Operation of the Poor Laws, England's poor law reform effort.[43] Chadwick, who was scientifically minded, compiled data from around the country on diseases, birth and mortality rates, and poverty rates, and he made important connections between poverty, overcrowded housing, sanitation, and poor health. Chadwick's report to the royal commission led to the 1834 Poor Law Amendment Act. This new Poor Law took away local and parish control for poor taxes and the care of paupers, establishing instead a national-ized and centrally administered system under the control of the London-based Poor Law Commission, led by physicians. The re-forms called for a reduction in "outdoor relief," meaning mon-etary and bread rations given to individuals and families living in their own housing. Instead, the law called for an increase in "indoor relief," forced entry into institutions, usually in the form of workhouses. Chadwick's "workhouse test" was that these in-stitutions were meant to be more economical and to be much more unpleasant than outdoor relief. Workhouses were austere, unpleasant places of last resort for poor people. They included mandatory work requirements, the wearing of uniforms by all paupers, the forced separation of couples and families by age and gender, and severe food rationing. In effect, workhouses were so-cial experiments that were essentially prisons to punish people for being poor.[44] This was the case in America, reputedly the land of unlimited opportunity and social class leveling, as in England. The workhouse or poorhouse was designed to be the "ultimate defense against the erosion of the work ethic in early industrial America."[45]

By the middle of the nineteenth century in both Britain and America, the treatment of poor people was increasingly im-pacted by scientific discoveries, public health interventions, the rising prestige of physicians, and through the work of Florence Nightingale, the increased standards for and use of nurses. There was a greater emphasis on cost containment, surveillance of the poor and homeless, and greater governmental and social control of every aspect of their lives. It was thought that charity work should be organized along scientific lines, made more efficient, empirical, rational, and secular—what has come to be known as "scientific charity."[46] This surveillance of the poor extended to include the well-founded fear by poor people that their bodies were not their own in life or in death. Paupers could be experimented on in the name of science during their lives through the social experiment of scientific charity, or as medical specimens of disease and deformity, and after death through dissection of their bodies.

England, Scotland, and US states such as Massachusetts, New York, Pennsylvania, and Maryland, which had early medical schools, had only allowed dissection of the human bodies of criminals, both male and female, who were condemned to hang, and dissection was included as an explicit part of their punishment by many judges. To most people, dissection was a fate worse than death.[47] The pervasive Christian belief at the time, held by both Catholics and Protestants, was that resurrection required an intact and properly buried body with a Christian service. Cadavers dissected for medical science could not be resurrected, and so criminals were denied a Christian burial. Hangings began to taper off while university medical schools grew, so there was a shortage of cadavers. This led to an illegal trade in dead bodies, including recently buried corpses, which were regularly exhumed and sold to medical schools by the body snatchers.[48] Teeth were removed from the cadavers and sold to dentists for the making and selling of dentures.

There were cases, such as the highly publicized William Burke and William Hare trial of 1828 in Edinburgh, of outright murder in order to profit from the sale of bodies, especially of insane, homeless, or impoverished people in crowded areas of cities, like Old Town in Edinburgh or London. At the time, Edinburgh had the leading medical school in the world. Most of the sixteen confirmed victims of Burke and Hare were poor and Irish, and many were women, including prostitutes the two murderers felt no one would miss. One of their victims who was missed by many townsfolk was known as "Daft Jamie." James Wilson was an eighteen-year-old "rough sleeper" and beggar in Edinburgh who was mentally ill or developmentally disabled and had a deformed foot. He was a familiar figure on the streets of Old Town, and his cadaver was easily identified by the police.

The British passed the Anatomy Act in 1832 to try and address the issue of body snatchers, also known as resurrection men. The new Poor Laws of 1834 included provisions for people forced into workhouses who died there and whose relatives did not claim and pay for the body within seven days. In such cases, the overseers of the poor in the workhouses could sell the bodies to medical schools and keep the profit.[49] William Cobbett, a British Parliament member and an outspoken critic of the new Poor Laws, stated, "They tell us it was necessary for the purposes of science. Science? Why, who is science for? Not for poor people. Then if it be necessary for the purposes of science, let them have the bodies of the rich, for whose benefit science is cultivated." He suggested that members of the royal family offer their bodies for science.[50]

In America, individual states developed their own anatomy laws and modified them in the early nineteenth century largely along the lines of the English Anatomy Act and the new Poor Laws. American medical schools, especially in the northeastern seaboard states, were growing and so was their need for sufficient numbers of cadavers. This led to grave robbing, including directly by medical students themselves. A cemetery for free Black people in New York City was frequently the site of body snatching as were cemeteries for Irish Catholic immigrants.[51] The new anatomy laws of states like New York, Massachusetts, and Pennsylvania made it legal to sell and dissect the bodies of paupers from almshouses. The US anatomy laws, like the ones in England on which they were modeled, were designed to be deterrents to and punishment for pauperism.[52] Inequality and structural violence in society extended into and even past death.[53]

Though there were no medical schools yet in the area, people in Seattle, including the poor and homeless, would have known about body snatching and what was being done at the time in other American cities about the dissection of paupers. Most of the poor patients who died at the Poor Farm and Hospital were buried in unmarked graves in the paupers' cemetery, Potter's Field, located there. This practice continued until 1912 when the King County commissioners had a crematorium built at the poor farm site, disinterred the bodies of 3,260 paupers, and cremated them.[54] Very poor records had been kept of the identities of the poor people buried in Potter's Field. Of the 3,260 bodies exhumed and then cremated at the King County Poor Farm and Hospital, 850 had names and dates of death, 493 had only patient numbers, and the remaining bodies had no identifying records. One of the men involved with the exhumation and cremation of the county paupers reported that all their ashes were dumped in the nearby Duwamish River.[55]

Nurses were involved in Poor Law reform debates. After Florence Nightingale's work during the Crimean War, she established the London-based Nightingale Training School in 1860. The Bellevue Hospital Training School for Nurses, the first North American nursing school based on Nightingale's principles, opened in 1873 in New York City. The Quaker social reformers, the Rathbones of Liverpool, who also assisted Dorothea Dix with her mental health reform efforts in England and Scotland, asked Nightingale to introduce trained nurses into the British workhouse system, starting with the Liverpool Workhouse Infirmary in 1865.[56] This workhouse was reputed to have turned into the largest brothel in England, and its cohort of slatternly, alcoholic nurses was a disgrace.

With Nightingale's assistance, the Rathbones also hired well-trained nurses to do home visits with poor people, especially with poor families. Their nursing role included care for the sick and injured, but also lessons in hygiene and moral admonishments to practice temperance, thrift, limitations on family size, and hard work. In effect, nurses became agents of social control and part of the surveillance of scientific charity. Florence Nightingale called for more nurses to come from middle-class backgrounds versus working-class ones since she believed that higher-class women were more intelligent and could provide better moral uplift to downtrodden and immoral paupers. As Nightingale wrote in an influential letter to the *Times* on Good Friday, April 14, 1876, with the title "On Trained Nursing for the Sick Poor," such trained nurses from "a higher stamp of woman" depauperized people. The term "depauperized" was used in a similar fashion to "decontaminate" or "delouse."[57]

Charles Dickens, whose descriptions of untrained nurses in workhouses include the infamous character Sarah Gamp in his 1842 novel, *Martin Chuzzlewit*, worked with Florence Nightingale on the Committee of the Association for Improving Workhouse Infirmaries. As a child, Dickens's father had been sent to the Marshalsea debtor's prison in London. Dickens lived in a rooming house next to the Cleveland Street Workhouse as a boy and again as a young man during the years he wrote *Oliver Twist; or, The Parish Boy's Progress* (1839). In Dickens's novel, Oliver is born in a London workhouse to an unmarried woman who dies soon after childbirth, and the disheveled, tippling midwife steals her jewelry. Dickens makes clear to his readers that the body was then sold to anatomists, since Oliver's mother does not have a grave.

Dickens's novels were widely popular in America and were circulating among women settlers in the early days of Seattle. By that time, Dickens had written and published not only *Oliver Twist*, but also *David Copperfield* (1850), *Bleak House* (1853), and *Hard Times* (1854). His writing helped sway public opinion in both England and America against the overly harsh realities of the workhouse and the criminalization of poverty. Nevertheless, workhouses continued to exist in England and in places in America, especially in southern states, well into the twentieth century, after which many in the United States were turned into old age homes—and in England into public hospitals for what became the National Health Service. Dickens founded Urania Cottage in London in 1847. He called it simply "the Home," and it was a refuge and rehabilitation and education site for "fallen" girls and women prostitutes.[58] Dickens interviewed the young girls at the Home and took notes on their life histories, which he then used as source material for his books. This practice has been called "benevolent stalking."[59] Ostensibly, the purpose was to "rehabilitate" the girls and send them to the British colonies to work as domestic servants. Young girls in domestic service in London were particularly at risk of being caught up in the life of prostitution to support themselves and often to support their impoverished families. In both England and America at the time, the main source of social welfare for women was marriage, but that only worked for middle-class women.

■ ■ ■

After a year at the King County Poor Farm and Hospital location in what is now Georgetown, the Sisters of Charity of Providence appealed to Mother Joseph, who in the summer of 1878 visited Seattle from Vancouver and agreed that they needed to relocate their hospital to Seattle. Mother Joseph spent several weeks in the city visiting different locations and finally purchased the Moss Residence at the corner of Fifth and Madison Streets in the center of Seattle. She then drew up plans for remodeling the house to serve as their new hospital and supervised the construction. The three local Sisters, along with their four patients, moved into the new hospital on July 27, 1878.[60] The new hospital could accommodate thirty-five patients as well as the Sisters.[61] After the move, the Sisters began to do home visits with poor patients and families in addition to their hospital work. They had a designated "night nurse" to provide home care for dying people. This grew to include the work of lay Catholic women in their Ladies of Charity program.[62] Wanting to remove the stigma of the poorhouse designation from the hospital, the Sisters renamed it Providence Hospital.

Despite their move to a central location in Seattle and changing their name to Providence Hospital, however, the Sisters record in the *Chronicles* that they continued to have difficulties both in attracting patients and in what they termed the "injustice" of religious bigotry toward them by citizens of Seattle and by city and county officials. The perceived injustices included having their hospital quarantined, first for typhoid, then cholera, and later for a smallpox outbreak. They continued to have high death rates at the hospital, which did not help their reputation. In addition, many Seattle residents claimed they only attracted patients who wanted the large quantities of liquor the Sisters dispensed as medicine. Indeed, a review of the meticulous expense ledgers kept by the Sisters during this time shows frequent purchases of "liquor and spirits" as well as funeral shrouds, chicken feed, groceries, and coal.[63]

Early on the cold morning of Wednesday, November 5, 1879, a Seattle policeman knocked on the door of Providence Hospital and handed over a wooden box containing a newborn baby to the shocked Sisters. The baby was wrapped in bloody and stinking rags, was pale and blue, and appeared to be dead. Chief of Police Thorndike assured them that he had noticed signs of life in the infant, so they placed the baby beside the stove, carefully unwrapped the tiny body, and gave the boy warm baths until he revived.[64] They quickly had him baptized and named him Joseph after one of their favorite patron saints. A physician cut and tied the umbilical cord. Chief Thorndike, alerted by a resident who had heard the baby's weak cries, had discovered Joseph at the bottom of an outdoor latrine on Third Street near the intersection with Madison Street and close to the First Presbyterian Church. Thorndike traced a woman's boot prints from the privy through the alleyway and up toward the Territorial University.

Using the boot prints, as well as a piece of a child's flannel clothing found with the infant, Thorndike soon found the baby's mother. She was Mary Tucker, who had been among the Sisters' earliest patients at the King County Poor Farm and Hospital and was now a twenty-one-year-old "quadroon girl" working for the Post family as a servant. Tucker was taken to Providence Hospital where she identified the father of her infant, whom the Sisters recorded as being a "well-known logger from Skagit County."[65] The father must have had the last name Britton since the Sisters listed both Mary and Joseph with that surname instead of Tucker. The implication in the *Chronicles* and various newspaper accounts is that Mary Tucker had been supplementing her work as a servant with work as a prostitute. In the patient ledger, the Sisters claim Joseph as a Catholic, while his mother is listed as Protestant. Joseph is listed as "mulatto" and Mary as "mulatta."[66] Tucker told police he was born around five o'clock in the morning in the latrine behind the house where she had been employed as a servant for the past four months. She had effectively hidden her pregnancy from her employers and resumed her usual household duties right after giving birth in the outhouse.

The *Daily Intelligencer* article on Saturday, November 8, 1879, titled "Baby Mystery Solved" states that when asked why she abandoned the baby, she "said she was afraid of being discharged from her situation, and would have no place to go." What had happened to her previous baby, John Tucker, who would have been two years old, is not mentioned in any of the newspaper reports nor by the Sisters, who should have remembered both him and Mary Tucker from their earlier hospital admissions. Tucker stayed with her infant, Joseph, in the hospital and breast-fed him. Townsfolk brought presents for the baby. Tucker was facing likely prison time for attempted infanticide, in which case her infant son would go to prison with her. The Sisters told the police they would keep both Tucker and her baby in their care until a suitable work position opened for Tucker where she could either keep Joseph with her or find a family to foster and perhaps adopt him. There were no foundling hospitals or orphanages in Seattle at that time.

On November 27, Mary Tucker and infant Joseph were still patients at Providence Hospital. The Sisters conducted a fund-raising bazaar in Seattle that day and checked on their patients when they returned to the hospital in the evening, but the next morning they discovered that Tucker and her baby were gone. One Seattle paper reported that the two had taken a night boat to Victoria, British Columbia, and that "a sigh of relief went up all around. We had had enough and more than enough of the affair, and the more we had of it the more the name of our town and the people [were] smirched and soiled."[67] If she actually had gone to Canada, Mary Tucker likely would have changed her name to avoid being discovered and brought back to Seattle to face charges. However, a summary of events surrounding her that was recorded in the *Chronicles* states that Tucker and her baby were apprehended by Seattle police, brought back to town, and then sent to California to live.[68]

This was a high-profile case that turned public sentiment against Mary Tucker, an "abnormal" and "inhuman" mother. Tucker was described as stupid, but also as a victim of the baby's father, who cast her aside. No one seems to have mentioned that there were extremely limited options for an unmarried, uneducated young woman like Tucker, especially for a mixed-race woman. The case of "Baby Boy Britton" helped boost the reputation of the Sisters and their work, at least for a while. Public opinion changed in their favor, and the King County commissioners extended their contract for the nursing and medical care of the county poor. Later, when the Sisters ran short of money to pay their county taxes, the tax bill mysteriously disappeared. Changes to US tax laws giving exemptions to faith-based hospitals, including the extensive network of Catholic hospitals, did not occur until the 1940s.[69]

■ ■ ■

Much of what has been written about the work of the Sisters of Charity of Providence could be viewed as Catholic propaganda since it is authored by Catholics and published by Catholic entities. At the same time, the importance of their work cannot be dismissed. Whatever their motivations, most of the work of the Sisters of Charity of Providence clearly was done with compassion. It was their version and understanding of Christian charity. Catholic Sisters across America did so much more in terms of hospital building and administration than any other group of women at the time could. Through their role as "humble and gracious nuns, they could obtain certain courtesies or refuse secular direction without being seen as prideful or rebellious."[70] The Sisters of Charity of Providence used this to their advantage in their medical work in Seattle.

The King County commissioners began to feel pressure to have a better separation of church and state as they considered further renewals of their contract with the Sisters of Charity of Providence for their care of ill paupers who were wards of the county. An outspoken critic of the Sisters and their hospital was the influential Reverend Jacob F. Ellis, minister at Plymouth Church, located near the Territorial University in Seattle. A published synopsis of a sermon he preached on the topic begins, "Providence Hospital makes its appeal on the score of charity." Rev. Ellis states that King County was paying the Sisters 87.5 cents per patient per day for work that "is done elsewhere for 25 cents" and that by the end of their current five-year contract, the county will have paid them "$16,241.80, an amount of money sufficient to pay for the Hospital grounds and buildings, and put a handsome profit in the Church coffers." He ends with "Providence Hospital is not a charitable institution and should not receive public patronage."[71] Father Francis Xavier Prefontaine, a Catholic priest in Seattle, countered that the Sisters were "animated by true Christian charity" and that "the prosperity of this city is due to the liberality and charity of its people." He ended his letter to the editor with "Mr. Ellis, mind your own business and you will be a better man."[72] It is interesting to note that Father Prefontaine was a secular priest, meaning he had not taken a vow of poverty. During his long career in Seattle he accumulated significant property holdings, he was fond of fine whiskey and cigars, and he died a rich man.[73] In their *Chronicles*, the Sisters record this episode under the heading "Injustice," stating that it was further proof of testing by the devil.[74]

The King County commissioners were feeling pressure to not use public funds from taxation to pay a religious order, even if it was to contract out the care of ill paupers. It is likely they also wanted more direct control over the cost of care, which was rising. Male physicians likely wanted control over the county hospital since the Sisters, who were nurses, wielded considerable power under the current arrangement. As a result, the commissioners expanded the hospital facility at the original Poor Farm and Hospital in Georgetown and on February 1, 1887, the twenty-eight county patients under the care of the Sisters were transferred to the King County Hospital in Georgetown. Charles H. Merrick, a former Union Army physician, was paid $900 a year by King County to provide medical care to ill and injured indigent residents.[75] His wife (her name is not recorded) became the matron of the hospital, and they employed nurses to provide care. In their *Chronicles*, the Sisters lament the loss of these county patients, who now would be cared for by infidels—Protestants.[76]

4

ARK OF REFUGE

Mere charity only bails the boat and justice alone will stop the leak.
—Malcolm McDonald, "The Samaritan Spirit—Seattle's Pharisees"

On a breezy, cool morning in early June 1900, a bearded man wearing a dark suit and a black derby hat stood on the top deck of the side-wheeler *Idaho* gazing at the bustling Seattle waterfront. The tide was high, but the aged 174-foot former opium-smuggling boat was decommissioned, positioned on a gridiron, and not affected by the tides. Its mooring was along the city dock, built out from the sawdust-filled area at the foot of Jackson Street near where Madame Damnable's hotel and the Maynards' Seattle Hospital had stood. These wood structures, Yesler's dock, and even some of the sawdust had burned the decade before in Seattle's Great Fire. But in its wake, with a combination of investment money and the contagious city pride termed the "Seattle spirit," most of downtown, including Skid Road and the docks, had been rebuilt. Now, the odors of acrid coal and wood smoke, hay-sweet hops from a nearby brewery, foul rot from piles of garbage, and the ever-present fish, fir resin, and creosote permeated the air. A large warehouse of Terminal C, the Pacific Coast

Building, loomed beside the man. In front of him were the tracks of the Northern Pacific Railway, which finally connected Seattle with the rest of the country. Railroad Avenue, now Alaskan Way, at the time had eight railroad tracks on a 120-foot right-of-way that was built of wood planks on elevated trestles above the Seattle waterfront. Horse-drawn delivery carts could be seen beside freight and passenger trains. A wood gangplank connected the boat to the wharf. The man watched as several young workers from the *Idaho* rolled wheelbarrows down the gangplank, across the railroad tracks, and into the heart of Skid Road. On the front of the boat's engine room was a hand-painted wood sign proclaiming Wayside Mission Hospital.

Dr. Alexander de Soto had finished his morning devotional, checked on patients in the general ward, touched base with the two nurses—thirty-one-year-old hospital matron Irene Byers and eighteen-year-old Georgia Davidson—and prepared to walk the streets of the White Chapel area of Skid Road near where the hospital boat was moored. On these walks, de Soto engaged in conversations with chronic inebriates, prostitutes, people addicted to cocaine, morphine, and opium, railroad hobos, homeless drifters, and anyone else who might need free medical care, a meal—and spiritual salvation.

The Seattle police brought such people to the Wayside Mission Hospital. Those who were injured in their work along the bustling docks and streets of Seattle, as well as pedestrians harmed when crossing the dangerous Railroad Avenue while inebriated, found themselves as patients in this hospital. Wayside was the only emergency hospital in the burgeoning town. Providence Hospital and Seattle General Hospital had no emergency centers, and King County Hospital was still located south of town on the old Poor Farm and Hospital grounds in Georgetown along the Duwamish River. The men with wheelbarrows from the *Idaho* made daily rounds along the waterfront and collected donated fish, fruit, and vegetables for the shipboard cook to use for feeding patients, hospital staff, and homeless people, who were given free meal tickets by the mission staff. De Soto, almost sixty years old and seemingly a single man at the time, lived in a former stateroom on the boat, next to the free dispensary. A Seattle magazine's photograph of his shipboard bedroom shows a simple iron-frame bed covered with white linens, a large wood cross on the wall above the bed, and on the bedside tables, an open leather-bound Bible, a photograph of Chief Joseph, a human scapula, and a human skull. The skull holds pencils in the eye sockets.[1]

Short of stature and tall of tales, de Soto was by some accounts a highly educated, skilled, compassionate physician and surgeon, and by other accounts a charlatan, medical quack, faith healer, quixotic dreamer, and con artist. Born on July 24, 1840, in the Canary Islands to the Spaniard Alexander de Soto and the American Elizabeth Crane, Dr. de Soto claimed to be a direct descendant of the sixteenth-century Spanish gold seeker and explorer Hernando de Soto. He told people that as a young man in Spain he had studied for the Jesuit priesthood, fell out with the Catholic Church, became an agnostic, and then completed his education at the University of Madrid. In several reports, he claimed to have been a member of the Don Carlos movement in Spain and that he swam across the harbor of Calais to escape capture and climbed aboard a British merchant vessel.[2]

In 1862, de Soto migrated to New York City where it does not appear that he tried to practice medicine of either the faith-based or conventional sort. Instead, according to his own reports, he became a professional gambler and a morphine addict; was a US Navy captain in the War of the Pacific; traveled to Central America and Denver, Colorado, where he worked in mines; fought in various "Indian wars" in the American West; and then returned to New York City with even worse morphine and gambling addictions. He lived in tenements, police station homeless shelters, and on the streets in the Mulberry Bend area of lower Manhattan. De Soto cured himself of his addictions—if not his wander-lust and fondness for embellished stories—in 1890 through the Holiness movement at the Bowery Street Mission, one of the first such missions in the country.[3]

The Holiness movement, an outgrowth mainly of the Method-ist Church, was an evangelical part of the Third Great Awakening in America. Methodism had its roots in England beginning in the eighteenth century and quickly spread to the United States, maintaining a strong identification with the working class. Methodists eschewed higher education for their clergy and sup-ported itinerant lay preachers who advocated for direct charity and social reforms that included temperance, fair wages, better working conditions, women's suffrage, and anti-prostitution ef-forts. William Booth, a Methodist minister, and his wife, Cath-erine, established the Salvation Army in London's impoverished East End. The official motto of the Salvation Army was "Heart to God, Hand to Man," emphasizing personalized, hands-on, direct service and charity work.[4] Booth advocated for the spreading of the gospel through "slum sisters," unmarried women serving in pairs, living and working in impoverished urban areas, visiting and providing health education and care to poor families. The slum sisters were an early form of both social work and district nursing.[5] The Salvation Army spread throughout "darkest Eng-land" and then to the United States and many other countries.

A curious phenomenon developed in these evangelical move-ments with an unspoken belief along the lines of the more you have sinned, the farther you have fallen off the path of righ-teousness, the more impressive your salvation. A French histo-rian of England, Elie Halevy, claimed that Methodism offered a distraction from the deepening despair, hunger, and misery of poor people in rapidly industrializing England, and it was also a barrier to the propagation of revolutionary ideas that could lead to class warfare.[6] The Methodist Church provided sociopo-litical stability and a strong emphasis on British philanthropy by wealthy people for social and "scientific" charities directing services to the "worthy poor." The Holiness movement in America followed this pattern and included itinerant street evangelists and rescue missions for men and for "fallen" girls and women. These urban rescue missions had their beginnings in the 1870s in the slums and overcrowded tenement districts of New York City and Boston with their mostly poor European immigrants. Rescue missions then spread to other urban areas throughout the country.

■ ■ ■

The American Gilded Age, which featured railroad, oil, coal, steel, industrial, and financial tycoons combined with weak governmental controls, had created large income inequities, social unrest, and an unstable economy. Proponents of social Darwinism believed in the survival of the fittest, which in this case they equated with the wealthiest; the poor should be left to die and go extinct. There were major US and European bank failures and market crashes, leading to widespread economic depressions, including a "long depression" in 1873–1879 and another in 1893. In response to the excesses and social injustices of the Gilded Age, the rise of the Progressive Era in the 1890s saw a focus on human rights, social reforms, and government control of monopolies. The Progressive Era extended to 1920 when white women finally won the right to vote through the Nineteenth Amendment.

During the Progressive Era, the Holiness movement combined with other mainly Protestant groups to form the Social Gospel movement with its emphasis on Christian ethics applied to sociopolitical problems. A Danish immigrant turned muckraking American journalist, Jacob Riis, while focusing on poverty in New York City, which he knew firsthand, brought to his middle-class audience a message of the necessity for enlightened self-interest. Using the recently developed field of statistics, Riis advocated for the halting of the spread by poor people of infectious disease, despair, crime—and, possibly, class warfare—through a combination of benevolence and municipal reforms.[7]

In his popular book *How the Other Half Lives* and his subsequent *The Children of the Poor*, in order to plead for reforms, Riis combined forceful prose, Bible quotes, and health statistics (including crude death and child mortality rates) with photographs of sweatshops and people living in squalid tenements, in police station homeless shelters, and on the streets.[8] His writing caught the attention of then New York City police commissioner and future US president Theodore Roosevelt, who walked into Riis's office one day and asked what he could do to help. With Roosevelt's assistance, Riis advocated for the closing of police lodging houses, pointing out that the police should not be in the business of homelessness. Instead, they opened a rooming house for up to 200 homeless men on a barge on the East River and then developed rooming houses on Henry Street near where a public health nurse and social reformer, Lillian Wald, was already running the successful Henry Street Settlement house. In *The Children of the Poor*, Riis claimed that the way to end the cycle of poverty was to focus on addressing child poverty. He called for an increase in the literal "farming out" of poor children to be fostered and adopted by western frontier farm and ranch families. He highlighted the work of the Fresh Air Fund, which sent urban poor children to the countryside and operated floating hospitals in New York City for babies and for poor patients with consumption.

Riis writes in his autobiography, *The Making of an American*, about his own period of homelessness as a young adult in the Mulberry Bend area of New York City.[9] He describes the frequent police violence toward homeless people, including an incident when a police officer beat to death Riis's dog—his only companion—in front of him. But as the title of his book suggests, Riis emphasizes his "becoming American" through individual hard work and thrift, feeding into the bootstrap American myth.

Riis's progressivism only went as far as calling attention to the dangers to US society of continued urban poverty. Riis advocated for Christian and scientific charity instead of government benefits, which he felt led people to expect assistance and created a class of lazy paupers, whom he called "tramps." He did not address larger, systemic sociopolitical inequities. There were, however, an increasing number of people in the United States calling for more radical systemic reforms.

The July 4, 1892, Omaha Platform of the newly formed National People's (Populist) Party called for enactment of a graduated federal income tax, an eight-hour workday, government ownership of the railroads, fair pensions for Union soldiers and sailors, fair and equitable land use policies, voting reforms, and the legislative system known as "initiative and referendum." This legislative system allows voters to propose and pass legislation directly instead of through elected officials. In 1912, Washington would become one of the first states to adopt initiative and referendum, a form of direct democracy that continues today and remains concentrated in western states. In the preamble of the Omaha Platform the People's (Populist) Party writers stated, "The fruits of the toil of millions are boldly stolen for the colossal fortunes of a few . . . and the possessors of those in turn despise the republic and endanger liberty. From the same great womb of governmental injustice we breed the two great classes—tramps and millionaires."[10]

Seattle, although growing in population, remained little more than a colonial western outpost town at the time of the national founding of the People's (Populist) Party. Seattle did not have any robber baron millionaires. Indeed, its richest person, Henry Yesler, died without a will in 1892, and his relatives were fighting over what was left of his wealth. These relatives included the twenty-two-year-old niece he had married after the death of his wife, Sarah. They did not include his daughter, Julia, presumably his only surviving offspring since his son and only child with

Sarah had died in childhood. Julia could not inherit from her father because she was illegitimate, born of his unofficial marriage to the teenage Susan, the daughter of a Duwamish chief. Although Seattle did not have millionaires at the time, in the eyes of many people the city did have more than its share of tramps, hobos, drifters, paupers, and other homeless people.

■ ■ ■

It is important to remember that from its founding, Seattle was built on logging, fishing, coal mining, and agricultural industries that relied on seasonal, low-skilled, manual, and mainly male workers. These industries went through boom-and-bust cycles mirroring national economic patterns. The working- and lower-class neighborhoods in Skid Road and Belltown swelled with out-of-work men in the winter months and during economic slumps. Cheap rooming houses—what would later be termed single room occupancy hotels—abounded, especially in the Skid Road area and along the waterfront. Shacks, like the one Angeline had lived in, were concentrated along the waterfront in Belltown and Skid Road. Residents of these shacks were widely and derisively known as "beachcombers."[11]

An influx of people to the Seattle area was made possible by the completion of the railroad to Tacoma, just south of Seattle, in 1883 and the Northern Pacific Railway finally making it to Seattle in 1893. Seattle's population rose exponentially from 3,553 in 1880 to 42,837 in 1890.[12] King County's population for that time period rose from 6,910 to 63,989. By 1900, Seattle's population had grown to 80,671 and King County's to 110,053. But during these years, at least two-thirds of the people in Seattle were passing through, looking for work—and a good time—and only stayed for a few years. During this period, Seattle likely had the nation's largest transient population.[13]

The original Poor Law of the Washington Territory, the 1854 pauper act invoked to care for Edward Moore, Seattle's first official pauper and homeless person, was reenacted in 1889 when Washington became a state. The one change legislators made was to open the possibility that cities could share in the responsibility of care for the indigent. Washington cities were authorized "to make any regulations necessary for the preservation of public morality, health, peace, and good order."[14] In 1893, with the national recession in full swing, Washington legislators passed a memorial motion on the "evil of pauper immigration."[15] Evidently, they were concerned about both an increase in "pauper dumping" and Washington State becoming a magnet for paupers to move to.

Among those moving to the Seattle area were recent European immigrants fleeing intolerable urban living conditions in places like New York City. Seattle mainly attracted what were then considered "good immigrants," meaning people from Norway, Sweden, and Germany who, even though their native language was not English, were white, Protestant, family-oriented, and hardworking.[16] Although Washington, as a territory and then as a state, never had overtly racist and discriminatory "Black laws" like neighboring Oregon, Idaho, and Montana, racism certainly existed. During the Civil War, Washington Territory's Republican Party came out against racial equality for African Americans, hoping to head off an influx of Black people moving from the South to the territory. Boosters, land promoters, and politicians continued to describe Washington as "the white man's country." The few African Americans who lived in Seattle were forced to work in menial, low-paying jobs as waiters, cooks, and railroad porters even if they were highly educated.[17] And women of all races were forced to rely on men for their support, whether through marriage or through prostitution. Only teaching and nursing were considered suitable professions for women.[18]

The building of the railroads in the Pacific Northwest also brought a significant population of Chinese men, who worked for low wages and thus, in the minds of working-class white men, suppressed wages and took their jobs. In Seattle, the Chinese lived in Skid Road along the waterfront. They were accused of immorality in "opium dens," of living in filthy conditions, of being—as Native Americans had been accused of being—vectors of disease, including smallpox and bubonic plague, and of illegally smuggling opium into the Pacific Northwest from China. The Port Townsend Custom House records show that the side-wheeler *Idaho* was indeed an opium-smuggling boat before it became the Wayside Mission Hospital. In just two months (December 1885 and January 1886), records show the seizure of 3,576 pounds of opium from the *Idaho* on its way to Seattle.[19]

The Knights of Labor, a national organized labor union active in the Seattle area in the 1800s, fomented race- and class-based anger, resulting in acts of violence against Chinese residents, including the infamous Seattle anti-Chinese riot of 1886. Under the pretense of public health and safety measures, a large group of Seattle residents, including many women, led by the Knights of Labor raided the homes of Chinese workers in Skid Road, forced the residents to flee to the nearby docks, and shipped at least 200 Chinese people to San Francisco. Many of the leaders of the riot then decamped to Port Angeles where they formed the Puget Sound Cooperative Colony, the first of Washington's many utopian groups built on socialist ideals aimed at improving the living conditions of the working class—albeit, mainly the white male working class.

Other utopian, back-to-the-land colonies were formed throughout the Puget Sound region. These included Equality and Freeland north of Seattle and Burley and Home to the south.[20] Equality, founded in 1897, had direct ties to the organizers of the national People's (Populist) Party. Their Brotherhood of the Cooperative Commonwealth planned to establish a socialist colony in a left-leaning state in order to convert the state and then the entire country to socialism. Washington State's third governor, John Rogers, a Seattle area druggist, was voted into office in

1897 on the People's (Populist) Party ticket. He not only openly welcomed cooperative communities, he even joined the Burley Colony.[21] In his 1897 pamphlet, *Free Land: The Remedy for Involuntary Poverty, Social Unrest and the Woes of Labor*, Rogers called for a return to the land, a homesteading, agrarian, arcadian reform, stating, "We claim our inheritance from Nature, the common mother of us all. A home for every family and a 'job' for every man is our demand."[22] He concluded, "Let us do this and the eyes of seventy millions of people inhabiting the United States will be turned to Washington, which will then be seen as the brilliant Star in the West, the brightest gem in the western sky."[23]

Middle-class, nonsocialist citizens of Washington cities, including Seattle, supported this back-to-the-land movement. In the view of historian Richard White, citizens "sought to make the cities a safer, more profitable, place for themselves by draining off the poor and discontented."[24] These urban boosters denounced the US Forest Service for wanting to reforest the by now considerable clear-cut areas, claiming that instead of trees the land should "grow men." The farms, most of which were located on nutrient-poor glacial till, failed. As White states, "The back-to-the-land movement in the Pacific Northwest produced neither trees nor men; instead, it perpetuated a cycle of human and environmental destruction."

The People's (Populist) Party in Washington advocated for a "single tax" (taxation based on land value and not on what workers produced), so it eschewed a state individual income tax, which to this day Washington State has never had. It also moved to abolish vagrancy laws, pointing out that these laws punished people for being poor.[25] Vagrancy laws, left over from the adoption of the old English Poor Laws aimed at punishing and "warning out" (moving along) poor people, were increasingly used throughout America, especially with the rising numbers of tramps and railroad hobos in the years following the Civil War. Washington State, specifically the Seattle area, was a magnet for idealists, for people not only wanting to reinvent themselves but also aiming to reinvent and improve US society.

■ ■ ■

Alexander de Soto was living and working at the Bowery Street Mission in New York when he caught gold fever during the Alaska-Yukon-Klondike gold rush. This was the gold rush announced to the world by the *Seattle Post-Intelligencer* on July 17, 1897, when the steamship *Portland* pulled into Seattle carrying "a ton of solid gold." Seattle boosters quickly capitalized on this event by advertising Seattle as the gateway to the Alaskan gold fields, as a city where prospectors could buy the mandatory one year's worth of supplies before shipping off to Alaska. Seattle was also a town with a wide-open vice section in Skid Road where men could have a good time celebrating their newfound wealth or, much more likely, drown their sorrows over their failure in the gold fields.

De Soto, who was calling himself Captain de Soto at the time, led a seven-man cross-country proselytizing expedition, setting out on foot from New York City to Seattle and hoping from there to take a boat to the gold fields in the Yukon. He planned to preach on the sins of greed and debauchery in Alaska—and, if he happened to find any gold himself, would put it all into his missionary work. He called the group of seven the Gospel Argonauts, and he appears to have relished publicity.[26] One of the men in his group had worked for the Barnum and Bailey circus as an advertiser. Another, George Garner, was a "short, stout Englishman," a former journeyman plasterer turned prizefighter, and a self-described "pauper drunkard" from the notorious Mulberry Bend area of New York City.[27]

The Gospel Argonauts planned to walk across the country, stopping to preach and take up collections to help pay their way. They left New York City in early November 1897 wearing heavy fur coats and carrying pickaxes, shovels, blanket rolls, a tent, and several rifles. They wore large silver crosses engraved with "R.L.B.M." for Rescue League, Bowery Mission. Newspapers in New York City, Washington, DC, and Wilmington, Delaware, ran articles about their expedition. In Wilmington's *Evening Journal*, de Soto added to his personal story by saying that because he had failed at first to heed the call of God to do mission work in the Klondike, "his children were taken away from him and his wife lost her reason."[28] He claimed that his wife was in an insane asylum. It is unclear exactly how far the Gospel Argonauts traveled on foot versus taking transcontinental passenger trains using money collected at their evangelical services. De Soto later said that they took the train from Omaha, Nebraska, to Seattle—presumably as paying passengers, although they just as likely could have ridden the rails for free as hobos.[29]

Upon his arrival in Seattle, likely in early June 1898, de Soto sought out local newspaper reporters to cover his missionary work and dreams. In a *Seattle-Post Intelligencer* article from June 30, 1898, titled "Klondike Evangelists," he called himself Captain Ferdinand de Soto, saying he had been a sea captain and claiming to have fought as a Union soldier in the Civil War with New York's Garibaldi Guard, a volunteer unit composed of various immigrant groups proving their patriotism and loyalty to their new country. In the article, de Soto announced that his Klondike gospel band would hold a service that evening at the First Methodist Church, the church founded in 1853 by David and Catharine Blaine. De Soto invited people to attend to learn more about his group's proposed missionary work.[30]

In early July, de Soto became sick with a recurring fever; it may have been malaria, a disease that remained prevalent throughout the frontier areas of the United States and in the southern states.[31] He convalesced in the dilapidated wood building of the former Grace Hospital, which had closed in 1893 and was now a rooming house and the site of the Mount Carmel Mission. Irving Safford, a young Associated Press reporter, visited and interviewed de Soto; he was led to the sick man's room by a young female nurse from the mission.[32]

In a half-page article titled "De Soto's Descendant and His Proposed Christian Work" in the *Seattle Post-Intelligencer* of July 31, 1898, Safford describes de Soto as "a little blue-shirted man" with "strong and shapely" hands, a "cultured Castilian accent," a "white, thin face" with delicate features," including "large and lustrous" eyes, a "mass of darkish hair," and "a fine, dark beard." Clearly smitten, Safford declares: "It is not often you see in a bearded man a face you may call only beautiful. Occasionally you see one, and it stays with you."

De Soto again refers to himself in this article as Captain Ferdinand de Soto, describes his earlier life, and in this version, claims to have married a famous New York City actress who died young, presumably of consumption. He has plans for a floating hospital he calls Christ Hospital, which he wants to have built in Seattle, transported to Dawson City, and established there as a mission hospital. He wants to raise $30,000 to do this. "The work, it needs me you know," he is quoted as saying, with a parenthetical addition by Safford—"he himself is a physician"—as if it just occurred to de Soto that he could claim to be a physician as well as a captain and a tragic widower.

The American West, after all, is full of people who reinvented themselves and changed their names, professions, and life stories. At that time throughout America, many people became physicians not through formal medical school training, but through apprenticeship and by simply presenting themselves as physicians. The regulation and licensing of medical practitioners was rudimentary at best even in older cities like New York. In Washington, which had only become a state late in 1889, physician licensing was just beginning.[33]

Once de Soto recovered from his illness, he decided to stay in the frontier city of Seattle, which was obviously in need of more Christian missionary and medical work. He began to present himself to townsfolk as Dr. Alexander de Soto. He moved into an abandoned barn in the Skid Road area along the tidal flats at the mouth of the Duwamish River. The barn, described in another newspaper article, was "without sign of bed or bench or stove or stick of furniture—utterly forlorn and forbidding."[34]

The tidal flats and wide mouth of the Duwamish River south of Jackson Street were being filled in by zealous city engineers; the winding Duwamish was straightened and dredged to enable the building of industries on the expanded flatlands. The marshy area of reclaimed land where de Soto lived in the barn was called White Chapel or the Lava Beds for its numerous brothels and rowdy saloons. Beginning in the 1880s with the town's population surge, this area was Seattle's first working-class neighborhood, along with the shantytown in Belltown where Kikisoblu lived and where she died in 1896.[35] From the barn, de Soto began a Robin Hood sort of medical practice. He charged high fees for medical consultations for rich people—especially rich women, who likely found him to be as beautiful and charming as Safford described—and then provided free medical care and food for the homeless and poor in Skid Road. Some of his homeless patients, likely including railroad hobos, lived with him in the barn.

By February 1899, de Soto had moved from the barn to a rented basement in a tenement building in the heart of Skid Road on Railroad Avenue between Main and Jackson Streets. He turned the basement into the Wayside Mission, presumably named for its location along the waterfront as well as for the mission's focus on services for people who had become society's castoffs and refuse. The Wayside Mission was "near the edge of the tide, that mysterious force that bears in and out, ceaselessly day by day, the flotsam and jetsam of human life," as one newspaper reporter put it.[36] He went on to say that "high tide or low tide, the neighborhood smells to heaven," since it is next to "the outlet of the city's sewers" and piles of rotting garbage "dumped on the streets." Skid Road, Yesler Way, had one of the city's first sewer lines installed. It ran beside the street, and, as logs had done in the early days of Seattle, the sewage ran downhill and dumped directly into Puget Sound.

In late June, Seattle newspapers announced the "Passion Play at the Jefferson Theater," which was a benefit for the Wayside Mission at fifty cents a seat.[37] "Dr. Alexander de Soto" was the lecturer. This is the first instance in print that he used the honorific for a physician. Soon after this benefit for the Wayside Mission, in early July, de Soto was back in the news, both locally and nationally, but this time it was for a story that he tried to suppress.

■ ■ ■

The headline of a July 3 *Seattle Post-Intelligencer* article about de Soto proclaimed, "Divine Healing Fails: Local Physicians Stirred Up by Death of Mrs. Karen Carlson: Blame Dr. Alexander De Soto."[38] An article in the Washington, DC, *Evening Times* of July 6 about this same event was titled "Didn't Pray Hard Enough: A Divine Healer's Excuse for a Sick Woman's Death."[39] De Soto had provided a home medical consultation to a Seattle woman who was having difficulty eating. He claimed that she asked him to pray with her during his visits and that this was the only care he offered except for prescribing medicated gargles to try to open her throat so she could swallow. He wrote "pharyngitis" (sore throat) as the cause of her death. He stated that he did not know that she had been under the care of Dr. Park Weed Willis for stomach cancer.

It is likely that the King County coroner and health officer only became involved in this case since Karen Carlson had been a wealthy and prominent citizen of Seattle. In addition, the group of regular physicians who brought this case to the attention of authorities were angry about what they saw as de Soto stealing a paying patient away from Willis, one of "their own," a regular physician who had been caring for Carlson. Of note, "regular physician" was a term used then to mean a biomedical doctor with a medical school education. Willis, a prominent Seattle physician and surgeon who had completed his medical education at the University of Pennsylvania, was the first president of the Washington State Medical Society and of the King County Medical Society. He was the nephew of Gideon A. Weed, Seattle's first health officer, enforcer of Seattle's ordinance on smallpox control, two-term Seattle mayor, and former co-worker of Doc Maynard at the Seattle Hospital. Willis came from a solid Seattle pioneer and pedigreed medical family.

The group of physicians accused de Soto of being a faith healer, a Christian Scientist, and not a "regular physician," and they pointed out that de Soto had no documented medical education. De Soto never had applied for a medical license in Washington State, likely because he knew he did not qualify for one. The physicians demanded that de Soto perform the official autopsy on Carlson with the King County coroner and their group members in attendance. De Soto refused, perhaps because he did not know how to perform surgery, much less an autopsy.

De Soto claimed that Park Weed Willis and the other physicians were picking on him because he was successfully caring for Seattle's "unfortunate souls" when they were not. He claimed to have provided free medical care to more than 1,400 patients. "It is my intention, if I can secure the means, to open a large free hospital and dispensary in this city both of which have been demonstrated are crying necessities," he told a reporter.[40] He threatened to move his medical mission to Alaska if he continued to be harassed in Seattle. It is interesting to note that this group of medical men apparently went on to tolerate de Soto's medical and surgical practice through the Wayside Mission Hospital, perhaps because it remained limited to "drug fiends," tramps, prostitutes, and paupers. A photograph of de Soto during a surgery at the Wayside Mission Hospital a few years later shows him administering a cloth with anesthesia, likely chloroform, with one hand and holding the patient's hand with the other. Two male surgeons operate on the patient while a young female nurse in a striped apron and white cap stands at the end of the operating table staring wide-eyed at the photographer.

■ ■ ■

The practice of medicine was undergoing massive changes with the rise of medical science, concentrated in Europe and England, and the work of Robert Koch, Louis Pasteur, and others identifying the causes of infectious diseases.[41] The germ theory was beginning to replace older theories of infectious disease, including the belief in miasma as the cause of illness. Florence Nightingale had believed in the miasma theory of disease and thus advocated general cleanliness, the draining of swamps and bogs, and the health benefits of living—or convalescing—high up on hills or mountains in fresh air.[42]

In the United States, there were only a few "regular" medical schools based on the newer discoveries of medical science, and they were concentrated on the East Coast. There were still large numbers of people, both men and women, claiming to be doctors of various sorts. Most were "irregular" or alternative health practitioners. Christian Science, founded by Mary Baker Eddy, by 1899 was well known but controversial. Eddy and her adherents believed in mental powers and prayer to cure illness. Hydrotherapy was popular, as were homeopathy, electrotherapy, diet fads, and general faith healing. It was common for people to bounce back and forth between regular and irregular doctors as they sought cures for their ailments. There was no regulation of the selling of self-made or patent medicines, and these could be purchased in drugstores or directly through the mail, which had become more efficient with the expansion of the railroads. Many of these patent medicines contained large percentages of alcohol, opium, or cocaine. They were widely popular as well as addicting and were used for babies as well as adults.[43]

Irregular doctors often were run out of areas, accused of being medical quacks, especially if one of their patients died under suspicious circumstances. Most irregular doctors were female, while the regular doctors were, for the most part, male since regular medical schools and societies barred women.[44] Many of the irregular doctors made their way west to less medically regulated locales.

The Pacific Northwest, for example, had the notorious Dr. Linda Burfield Hazzard, a diet and purging practitioner who was forced to leave Minneapolis before settling in Seattle and setting up her medical practice. Known as the "starvation doctor," she did succeed in getting a medical license from Washington State, but it was revoked after a sensational 1911–1912 trial accusing her of starving a British heiress to death, stealing her money, and selling her teeth for the making of dentures.[45] Hazzard also oversaw the "diet" of Norwegian immigrant and Seattle resident Daisy Haglund.[46] Haglund, who died of starvation at age thirty-eight, left behind a three-year-old son, Ivar, who later founded the restaurant Ivar's Acres of Clams on the Seattle waterfront. Hazzard was found guilty, had her medical license revoked, spent two years in Washington State's Walla Walla prison—and after release returned to her same medical work of dieting and purging. Hazzard preyed on gullible and desperate people of means and refused to care for anyone who could not pay her, either in life or in death.[47]

Soon after the controversy over the death of Karen Carlson, the Seattle health officer, Dr. M. E. A. McKechnie, placed de Soto and the residents of the tenement basement Wayside Mission under a fifteen-day quarantine for smallpox, stating that two of de Soto's mission patients had been diagnosed with smallpox the day before. The two patients were sent to the county pest house on the outskirts of town. McKechnie nailed a Keep Out sign to the front door of the mission and hung a yellow flag at the entrance—the sign of smallpox.[48]

De Soto protested, thinking, most likely, that this was continued harassment by the Seattle medical establishment, but he was forced to comply by a police officer stationed at the mission's doorway. Newspaper articles at that time routinely named the places and people under quarantine, especially if they fit the expected narrative of poor people and nonwhite people being vectors of disease. In this case, the *Seattle Post-Intelligencer* article of July 12, 1899, was titled "Twenty Men Locked in Wayside Mission Quarantined by Health Officer." The article describes how the Seattle health officer, the "city physician," and four police officers staked out the Wayside Mission the night before, waiting until "gray haired men" and "boys of 14" had gathered inside the basement mission for the 10:00 p.m. evening prayer service. The health officer and police then announced that the mission and all the men inside were under quarantine for smallpox for at least fifteen days with food to be provided at the city's expense. The two men with smallpox "were Charles Summerville and William Heath. Heath is a professional hobo and came from Montana, stopping at several towns on the way."

"Professional hobo" is an interesting way to describe William Heath. It implies that he was a longtime unemployed, homeless, and single man riding the railroads for free and traveling in search of temporary jobs. As such, he was part of a large, mobile, visibly poor, and homeless population of mostly white men, which had developed in America during the Gilded Age in the wake of the Civil War and with the expansion of the railroads. It has been suggested that Civil War veterans of both sides were so severely traumatized by the war and were suffering from what was then termed, ironically, "nostalgia" or homesickness and now termed post-traumatic stress disorder, that they were unable to reenter "normal" domesticated and family life. Of course, it did not help that the United States was rapidly industrializing and urbanizing, especially in the Northeast and Midwest, with industries relying on cheap, disposable workers. The men became used to riding the rails in search of jobs and living rough outside, so they became what was termed "tramps" and later "hobos."[49]

■ ■ ■

The journalist Jacob Riis, in addition to being homeless on the streets of New York City, took to the rails and was a tramp until landing his first newspaper job.[50] With the economic depression starting in 1873, thousands of unemployed men rode the rails in search of work. This population of homeless men led to the "tramp scare" with newspapers reporting how tramps highlighted "the struggles between the propertied and the unpropertied over the uses of public space, fears about the growth of a propertyless proletariat, and anxieties about the loss of traditional social controls in American cities."[51]

The tramp scare, also called the "tramp evil," grew in intensity during the 1880s and 1890s and continued at least until the US entrance into World War II. Stiffer anti-vagrancy laws known as Tramp Acts were put into place in New York in 1879, which allowed the immediate rounding up and imprisonment of anyone suspected of being a tramp or hobo.[52] The young, soon-to-be socialist, and famous American author Jack London, during his time of riding the rails, was imprisoned for a month in New York state under the Tramp Act.[53] Besides being denied a lawyer or any contact with friends or family members, he was "compulsorily vaccinated by a medical student who practiced on such as we."[54] London later attributed his turn toward socialism to this event. Tramps, more commonly called "bindle stiffs" in rural areas, were part of the migrant farm workers' flow up and down the West Coast, including into Washington. With the completion of the railroads and the increasing economic downturns in the national economy, hobos—professional or not—were an increasing presence in Seattle.

■ ■ ■

The smallpox quarantine at the Wayside Mission was followed by a Seattle municipal court case brought by Alexander de Soto against the landlady of the rooming house above his mission. He claimed that she was harassing him by stopping up her sinks and causing the basement mission to flood. She was fined ten dollars by the judge.[55] But the dousing occurred again later that year, and de Soto accused the same woman of pouring cold water through her floor onto a corpse—one of his homeless patients who had died and was in an open casket while they conducted his funeral service.[56] And, it should be noted, this patient's death was not investigated or questioned by authorities. Back in a Seattle court, the landlady, Mary Johnson, complained that "these people keep up a racket to all hours of the morning, and I can't keep my lodgers because they make such a noise about their religion."[57] De Soto's lawyer countered by exhorting the judge to "protect American citizens in their right to worship God according to the dictates of their own consciences."

In one of the more fanciful and overwrought Seattle news reports about the Wayside Mission work of de Soto, he is referred to as the Good Samaritan and is portrayed as a bearded and top-hat-wearing St. George helping the downtrodden and slaying the dragon of evil. De Soto and his mission workers are likened to Benedictine monks for "their life of poverty, privation, and risk of infection from disease."[58] The *Seattle Post-Intelligencer* reporter describes his visit to the mission at midnight when it is raining outside. The meal has been served, the evening devotional service has concluded, and fifty men are sleeping on canvas cots with quilts over them, their wet clothing and boots steaming in the warmth from a coal fire. The small kitchen has rough shelves, sides of bacon, and piles of vegetables. "Doctor Ferdinand De Soto" is in a back room tending to "a negro in the deliriums of fever" with "the soft, flexible, sure hands of the surgeon." De Soto's assistant, George Garner, the former prizefighter and Gospel Argonaut, describing their experiences with Christian salvation, points out to the reporter that de Soto "had so much farther to fall—his position being a physician—my own that of a laborer." Garner goes on to say that they charge five cents for a bed per night and five cents for a meal—although they waive the fee when needed. "We did not want men to feel they could get something for nothing. . . . That sort of thing pauperizes a man, makes him a tramp and a beggar," and this way "we keep the sting of having become a pauper from him." In an early form of harm reduction, they allow "drunkards, if not noisy or obstreperous," to have meals and stay the night. He estimates that one in twenty men is of the group "tramps and bums"; the other nineteen are temporarily out of work and seek the mission rather than sleeping "as a trespasser on the wharves in the cold and the rain." Seattle police regularly arrested and jailed people for vagrancy.

De Soto, the Good Samaritan, joined the First Methodist Church, where he met wealthy Seattle philanthropists and a Seattle judge who supported his idea of opening a hospital mission on a boat along the Seattle waterfront. They formed the Seattle Benevolent Society, convinced city officials to rent space to their association at the city dock, found and bought the decommissioned *Idaho*, and proceeded to convert the boat into a hospital. De Soto's idea for a floating hospital was not a novel one. He likely knew about and had seen the "fresh air" boats and floating hospitals for babies and for tuberculosis patients in New York City. And he may have known about Riis's barge that housed homeless people.

■ ■ ■

The Seattle Benevolent Society, composed of middle-class men and women, was one of an increasing number of organized charity associations in Seattle, many of them started and run by women. Henry Yesler's wife, Sarah, founded the first suffragist organization in Seattle and was one of the founders in 1884 of the Ladies Relief Society, Seattle's first benevolent association, which mainly assisted orphaned children. Throughout America, for middle-class and upper-class women, charity work became an index of social status. Newspapers in the late nineteenth century often listed their activities in the society pages.[59] Washington, while still a territory in 1883, granted women the right to vote only to have it taken away three years later through a technicality by the territorial Supreme Court. Also, it was taken away because women voters in Seattle effectively shut down saloons and places of prostitution, both of which were large sources of revenue for the city. Women's suffrage was left out of the constitution of the newly formed Washington State in 1889. But the state would bring back women's suffrage in 1910. Washington and other western states led the nation on this issue.[60]

Seattle women, especially once they regained the vote in 1910, impacted social and health policy at the local and state levels. Many of the Seattle area women's groups that focused on benevolence and social issues were at least nominally tied to various Protestant churches. As throughout the West, the Protestant churches put aside denominational differences and typically banded together around moral and social issues, including temperance and anti-prostitution efforts. The Protestant churches "became the leading institutions for shaping public morals in the West, but paradoxically, their public activities won them more influence than members."[61] Starting in 1910, two young Methodist deaconesses opened the Deaconess Settlement House in Rainier Valley for Italian immigrants. Jesse Gasser, a teacher, and Mary Jane Hepburn, a nurse, offered well-baby and nutrition clinics and evening English classes.[62] They conducted home visits along the lines of the public health work of the "Madonna of the Slums" in New York City, Lillian Wald.

Once Seattle women regained the vote, they banded together behind the widely popular—and populist—Presbyterian minister Mark Matthews in order to oust Seattle mayor Hiram Gill and to send his crooked chief of police, Charles "Wappy" Wappenstein, to prison for corruption and graft.[63] Wappenstein had been charging each of the estimated 500 Seattle prostitutes in the employment of two main vice leaders ten dollars a month in payoff.

The two vice leaders had been emboldened to form a corporation, the Hillside Improvement Company, and then obtained from the city council a fifteen-year lease on city land near the King County Poor Farm and Hospital and built a 500-room brothel. The exclusively male Clean City Organization and the Public Welfare League joined forces with Rev. Mark Matthews and with members of the General Federation of Women's Clubs to block the opening of this giant brothel.[64] The women plastered Seattle with flyers titled "An Appeal to Mothers and Fathers" and encouraged people to visit the half-completed brothel. The handbill concluded, "Let every mother and home-loving woman go to the polls on March 5 and vote for Mr. Cotterill so that these buildings may remain uninhabited: that our homes will remain unpolluted, and that the shame of Seattle may not be advertised to the world."[65] Women voters turned out in large numbers and helped George F. Cotterill to defeat Gill for mayor.

■ ■ ■

The opening of Wayside Mission Hospital in early April 1900 must have been an especially gratifying day for de Soto. A photograph of the event shows the old opium-smuggling boat the *Idaho* packed with more than a hundred men and women and a few children, all smiling for the camera. Many of the people photographed were members of the Seattle Benevolent Society. The heavily bearded Alexander de Soto stands by the boat's front railing.

The June 1900 US Census for Seattle's Precinct 1 in Skid Road records Alexander de Soto, physician, as head of the "household" of the Wayside Mission Hospital, accompanied by forty-nine "lodgers." Of the nine female lodgers, two are listed as nurses, including thirty-one-year-old Irene Byers, originally from Indiana. Dressmaker, servant, cook, and hairdresser are listed as professions for the other women. Among the men, there are seamen, lumbermen, carpenters, cooks, day laborers, a steamboat captain, a saloonkeeper, and a druggist. Everyone is recorded as being white except for Charles Chew, a forty-three-year-old cook who is listed as Chinese. De Soto's fellow Gospel Argonaut, the former prizefighter George Garner, is not included as a lodger, but he supposedly worked as the night watchman on the floating hospital.

In a late October 1900 newspaper article, de Soto is again described as having "soft, feminine, gentle hands."[66] The reporter adds that de Soto's detractors accuse him of having an "oriental imagination," emphasizing his exotic "otherness" and perhaps Moorish influence to the majority white Seattle population. But the reporter counters this otherness with the doctor's "systematic plan of applied Christianity," which has attracted many supporters of his mission work to provide medical care to those in need but "not to harbor 'hobos.'" He is described as a "practical mystic." De Soto tells the reporter that his biggest hurdle is finding appropriate homes and work for female patients "with records," presumably records of prostitution. De Soto hopes to provide training for them in burnt leather work and making children's clothing. He adds that some of the women apprentice as nurses at the floating hospital. "Their whereabouts will be kept secret and one by one their identity will be lost." The connotation here is that the women had worked in prostitution before becoming nurses and required assistance in assuming new identities. De Soto "attracts strong characters" to his work. One of those is Irene Byers. She is described as the main nurse and matron of the Wayside Mission Hospital; she received her nurse training from Seattle General Hospital and "could earn a good salary" but works for free. The reporter adds, "Recently Miss Byers took a much-needed vacation."

Besides finding support from Seattle benefactors, de Soto received funding directly from the city of Seattle for the care of patients addicted to morphine and of indigent patients. At the time, Seattle and King County had an agreement that the city would care for "ill paupers" if they had been in Washington State for less than six months.[67] In addition, the city agreed to take care of all emergency cases since the King County Poor Farm and Hospital was too far from the city and was not equipped for emergency care.

■ ■ ■

"An intractable cough!" is the opening sentence of a 1903 article in a national journal, the *Medical Bulletin*, written by Alexander de Soto and C. W. Crimpton of the Wayside Mission Hospital.[68] In this article, likely funded by the budding pharmaceutical industry, De Soto and Crimpton extol the virtues of a new cough medicine, glyco-heroin, produced by Smith Drug Company, then based in Philadelphia and now part of the multinational pharmaceutical giant GlaxoSmithKline. The recently formulated drug heroin was the medicine's main ingredient. Using language eerily similar to that used in the twenty-first century by pharmaceutical companies to extol the virtues of OxyContin, which led to the US national opioid epidemic, de Soto and Crimpton claim that this heroin-based product "is superior to morphine, and harmless." They include multiple case histories of patients who have been "cured" with the medication, including a twenty-two-year-old male with tuberculosis and a ten-month-old boy with a cough. They even treated the cough of a Seattle policeman.

One of the Seattle area's socialist newspapers, the *Commonwealth*, carried an article by Malcolm McDonald on May 23, 1903, titled "The Samaritan Spirit—Seattle's Pharisees." McDonald reports that the city wants to develop the land and dock where the Wayside Mission Hospital is located. But "it is the only hospital in the city ready at all times to receive the poor—the utterly poor who in sickness know no relief but death or the help of the Good Samaritan." McDonald points to the high commercial value of land along the Seattle waterfront and asks, "Is any land too valuable for the saving of a human life? Is there no room in Seattle for an institution that has pity and not profit for the motive of its existence?" The article is accompanied by photographs of the floating hospital, the "ark-of-refuge," including one of the dispensary next to de Soto's bedroom. The caption states, "Showing the free dispensary, where prescriptions are filled and all needed medicine supplied without prying into the deserving or undeserving character of the sick and poor." There is a sidebar photograph and story of a young Chinese woman identified only as Dora, a Seattle prostitute and "unpaid nurse" who cared for a dying "Klondike boy." "She did this when church ladies refused help."

In July 1904, de Soto was forced out of his work with the mission by the city and by members of the Seattle Benevolent Society because "his management became unsatisfactory."[69] The specific concerns are unclear. Was he keeping some of the donations to the mission hospital for his own private use, such as his purchase of a modest bungalow in Rainier Valley? Was the Seattle medical establishment deepening its concern over his lack of a "regular" medical background and his continued financial support from both the city and the county? Was he, as many driven and charismatic founders of such endeavors often are, overly self-identified with the Wayside Mission Hospital and not open to change? Or had it become more widely known that he had fathered a child in 1901 with his hospital matron, Irene Byers? Was the community concerned that he was living with her and their son, Alexander de Soto Jr., in his house in Seattle—but was not legally married to Byers? In an early and real-life version of a medical soap opera, their son was born May 20, 1901, in Santa Clara, California, likely when Byers took the "much needed vacation" from her work at the Wayside Mission Hospital.

Whatever the reasons for de Soto being forced out of the medical mission he had dreamed of, started, and run for four years, the floating hospital was turned over to Fanny W. Connor and Marion Baxter, benefactors and social reformers.[70] Under the leadership of these two women, the renamed Wayside Emergency Hospital continued to operate much as before on the *Idaho* along the Seattle waterfront.

■ ■ ■

Katharine Major, the nurse matron of the Wayside Emergency Hospital, was asked to write an article about the unique hospital by the editors of the recently established *American Journal of Nursing*. Major's article, "Nursing Seattle's Unfortunate Sick," appeared in the October 1905 edition.[71] In their comments, the editors describe their summer tour of the West Coast and visits to various hospitals. They deplore the conditions they found at the San Francisco County Hospital but praise the King County Hospital in Seattle as "an exceptionally comfortable institution—a good building, charmingly situated, with an atmosphere of cleanliness and sunshine everywhere."[72] They allude to also having visited other Seattle hospitals, which then included Providence Hospital and Seattle General Hospital. They claim that most hospitals they visited focused on profit. "We were told that the poor who applied for admission were sent to the county hospital—that there were no worthy poor on the Pacific Coast, that the man who had no money was either lazy or vicious." They comment on nursing on the West Coast as lacking the "vigor" of the East Coast with most nurses learning through apprenticeship instead of formal nursing education. They add that they heard complaints from Seattle nurses about paying patients like the ones at Seattle General Hospital who refused to be practiced on by novice doctors and nurses. The implication was that poor and homeless patients in hospitals like the Wayside Emergency Hospital and King County Hospital were the ones to practice on.

In her article, Katharine Major describes the work of the Wayside Emergency Hospital as "one of the most unique charities in the world," run on the principle of "Friend of the Homeless and Sick." The staff consists of six volunteer physicians and "eight carefully trained nurses whose training on the old ship has fitted them to compete with nurses of any other institution." She emphasizes that they perform some of the most "interesting and unusual operations known to surgery" and care for more than a hundred patients each month. She reports that most of their funding comes from private donations, but the city and county each provide $250 per month for the care of ill paupers. She declares that poverty or "the reckless, shameless life of others afford a city no excuse for carelessness and indifference" toward ill people. In a form of poverty tourism, she invites readers to stop by the hospital for a visit if they travel to Seattle.

In 1907, the *Idaho* became too leaky to repair, and they moved the Wayside Emergency Hospital to the Sarah B. Yesler Building, a former rooming house for working young women to help keep them away from the lure of prostitution. The Wayside Emergency Hospital continued to function until 1909 when Seattle opened its own clinic and hospital downtown on at Fifth Avenue and Yesler Way in the Public Safety Building. On the last day of

March 1909, nineteen patients were moved from the Wayside Hospital to the new Seattle City Hospital on the fourth floor of the Public Safety Building.[73]

■ ■ ■

After de Soto was forced to resign from the Wayside Mission Hospital, he continued to work as a physician in Seattle, but he largely disappeared from the news. He consulted on the leprosy case of a Seattle jail patient in January 1905. In the 1910 US Census, he is listed as the head of household and working as a physician, living in a house on Lucille Street in South Seattle with Irene; their son, Alexander de Soto Jr.; and their seven-month-old daughter, Ruth. That year, he ran for King County coroner on the Republican ticket but lost.

Alexander de Soto finally made it to Alaska and invested in gold and sulfur mines, as well as polar and grizzly bear furs. Commenting on de Soto's departure from Nome with his purchase of furs, the *Douglas Island News* reporter commented, "We shall probably hear from outside papers of the gallant doctor's hair-breadth 'scapes from the claws of the Kodiak Grizzly, the teeth of the mighty Polar Bear and the tusks of the man-eating walrus."[74] Curiously, the tall-tale-telling doctor reappears in a 1934 King County record. On January 13,1934—at age ninety-three—he married Irene. And the wedding was officiated by Rev. Mark Matthews at First Presbyterian Church in Seattle.[75]

There appear to be no additional US Census listings, public records, or newspaper articles about Alexander de Soto until November 12, 1936. In the *Brooklyn Daily Eagle* under the headline "Dr. De Soto, 96, Dies after Falling into Bay," de Soto is described as having been a dietician aboard the yacht the *Centaur*, which had just completed a tour of the Great Lakes and Florida.[76] "Dr. De Soto is said to have served the King of Norway as physician and dietician from 1910–1915." On the evening of November 11, de Soto lost his footing on the yacht's gangplank, was rescued by two sailors, but died of his injuries while in an ambulance on the way to a hospital. In his obituary, de Soto is described as "beloved husband of Irene De Soto of Seattle." The notice concludes with the parenthetical "Seattle, Washington, papers please copy." It does not appear, however, that any Seattle area papers ran this story.

Alexander de Soto and his Seattle waterfront floating mission hospital are much more than just quirky asides in the medical history and legacy of care for homeless people in Seattle. The Gospel Argonaut, the Good Samaritan, the practical mystic, through his medical mission work forced the citizens of Seattle not only to confront the reality of an increasing number of ill homeless people in their midst, but also to find innovative solutions for their care.

5

SHACKTOWN

Those people were my people. I respected them,
and the neighborhood was home to me.
—Hazel Wolf quoted in Susan Starbuck,
Hazel Wolf: Fighting the Establishment

Across from the Cadillac Hotel on Jackson Street in the heart of
Skid Road, a line of people snaked around the Seattle welfare office and into an alleyway of overflowing garbage cans and dark,
ice-slicked puddles. The sleet turned to fine mist on this Friday
morning in mid-December 1931. The effects of the stock market
crash of 1929, contributing to what became known as the Great
Depression, swelled the welfare, charity, and bread lines across
the nation. In Washington State, including Seattle, the anti-
quated Poor Laws were inadequate to care for the growing number of indigent people. Wearing threadbare coats, many people
in line were coughing, including a thin woman with sharp, bird-
like features and short brown hair partially covered by a black
wool hat.

Hazel Wolf, a thirty-three-year-old single mother, was waiting for her weekly food voucher at the "zone," the common name

for the welfare office. Behind Wolf, at the end of the alleyway looking south, rose a haze of gray smoke from jury-rigged stovepipes on a jumble of shacks made of cast-off lumber and pieces of automobiles, corrugated tin, and cardboard. Hooverville, or at least Seattle's largest Hooverville at nine and a half acres, had been built beside the town's main garbage dump on the former Skinner and Eddy Shipyard between the railroad yards at the end of Railroad Avenue and Puget Sound. This was rare Seattle flatland where the mouth of the Duwamish River had been before mining engineers washed away a nearby hillside and sluiced it into the former estuary to create land for shipyards, industries, and what was then the world's largest man-made island, Harbor Island. Before being destroyed, the hillside had connected Beacon and Yesler Hills since the last Ice Age with its retreating glaciers. The cut-through sections now were prone to frequent landslides. On top of what remained of Yesler, also called Profanity Hill and later First Hill, was the recently built fifteen-story King County hospital, Harborview. Emergency and acute care indigent patients were treated at Harborview, while chronic care and elderly indigent patients still resided at the old King County Poor Farm along the Duwamish River. Wolf and her daughter, Nydia, had been living near Harborview Hospital on Profanity Hill at St. Theresa's women's shelter, part of St. Mark's Cathedral.

With the birth name Hazel Anna Cummings Anderson and the childhood nickname Leo, which reflected her fierce tomboy personality, Wolf was born and raised in Victoria, British Columbia, in a low-income shacktown area on the outskirts of the small waterfront city on Vancouver Island, fifty miles across the Salish Sea from Seattle. Her American-born mother, Nellie Frayne Anderson, with only a fourth-grade education, was widowed when Hazel was ten and supported her three children with a patchwork of low-paying jobs: a seamstress in a garment factory that made overalls, a maid scrubbing floors, and an informal, untrained home nurse. She took into their home female boarders, including prostitutes and show girls who worked at hotels in downtown Victoria. During and after the gold rush, Wolf's red-haired, blue-eyed mother worked as a show girl and singer in a box house saloon in Victoria. Later in life, Wolf stated, "Once or twice I was allowed to go up in the balcony. All the women there were prostitutes—not that I had to avoid prostitutes. It was just no place for a kid."[1]

Hazel Wolf's father, George William Cummings Anderson, was a Scottish seaman born in Gibraltar who had migrated to Canada; he was badly injured in a factory accident when Hazel was five years old. Permanently disabled, soon addicted to lauda-num (an opium derivative), and in a wheelchair until he died, her father received no worker's compensation, so his wife supported the entire family. Wolf described her parents as atheists and so-cialists, and her mother was secretary of the local unit of the Industrial Workers of the World (IWW), known as the Wobblies, while working in the garment factory for three years. Hazel, be-tween the ages of seven and ten, would accompany her mother to IWW meetings.[2] "You might say I imbibed my desire to fight the Establishment with my mother's milk," Wolf would write in a letter to Dave Brower, first executive director of the Sierra Club, much later in her life.[3]

The IWW, begun in Chicago in 1905, quickly spread across the United States and into Canada; it advocated for "one big union" to replace the craft unions, such as the American Federation of Labor, which had replaced the Knights of Labor. The IWW em-braced a form of revolutionary industrial unionism with social-ist and anarchist roots and was especially strong in the Pacific Northwest among mining, timber, agricultural, and shipping workers.[4]

In early February 1919, the IWW joined a Seattle strike at the Skinner and Eddy Shipyard and helped to create a peaceful six-day solidarity general strike. Downtown Seattle was hushed and shuttered; even the streetcars ceased operation. The Seattle General Strike remains one of the largest and longest-lasting urban general strikes in the United States. Of course, the Labor Management Relations Act of 1947, known as the Taft-Hartley Act, later made general or solidarity strikes illegal and significantly undermined the power of labor unions. The Seattle strikers did not win any major concessions from industries, and Mayor Ole Thorsteinsson Hanson of Seattle proclaimed that he had helped defeat a Bolshevik revolution in the United States. The Russian Revolution of 1917 and the end of World War I late in 1918 had created a nativist backlash and a red scare throughout the United States. Immediately after the Seattle General Strike, Mayor Hanson ordered the arrests of leaders of the Seattle IWW and the Socialist Party, as well as the closing of the labor-owned daily newspaper, the *Union Record*.

In the aftermath of World War I, the Pacific Northwest experienced an economic slump. Seattle industries like the Skinner and Eddy Shipyard lost federal contracts, laid off workers, and soon closed. Wolf, who was now a single mother after a brief marriage, was living with her mother and infant daughter in the shacktown area of Victoria where she had been raised. Wolf had been forced by economic necessity to drop out of school after the eighth grade to work as a secretary to help her mother and two younger siblings financially.

As an older woman reflecting on this time of her life, Hazel Wolf described her bouts of depression, including what now would be termed a severe postpartum depression. With lifelong Christian Scientist leanings, Wolf claimed to have realized that the moods and depressive episodes "were physical, purely physical, based on some laws I didn't understand, like the cycles of the sun or the moon . . . so when the depressions would come, I'd talk myself out of them."[5] Wolf's lifelong tendency to outward activity and use of relentless humor and what she called one-line "zingers" may reflect coping mechanisms for her underlying depression. Telling an interviewer about her keeping and then destroying personal journals, Wolf stated, "I didn't want anyone prying into my mind."[6]

Wolf attempted to enter nursing school in Victoria but was turned away because it would not accept single mothers. Knowing that there were more job opportunities for women in Seattle, she moved to the city in 1923, leaving Nydia with her mother so that she could compete better in the job and housing markets. Later in life, Wolf talked about how much she loved the impoverished community in Victoria where she was raised. She had dreamed of becoming a doctor, nurse, social worker, or architect and returning there to provide health, social support, and improved housing for the people in that shacktown area. She grew up, in her own words, "class conscious. I knew we were poor."[7] Before he died, her father taught her "that the middle class stood as a buffer between the very poor and the very rich, and I didn't like the middle class. . . . I never knew I was going to grow up and be one. Even now I speak middle-class language with an accent because this is not my true world."

Safe, affordable housing in Seattle, especially for low-income single mothers like Wolf, was difficult to find. The shipbuilding industry, which had grown rapidly during World War I and recruited more than 20,000 men and, in many cases, their families from other parts of the country, stressed an already tight housing market.[8] Rooming houses and low-income hotels continued to be concentrated in the Skid Road area of Seattle. The missions in Skid Road were for men. Shacktown areas, such as the one in Belltown where Angeline had lived, still existed and grew considerably in the interwar years of the Great Depression.

In a 1932 essay originally titled "Women on the Breadlines," the formerly homeless single mother Meridel Le Sueur wrote about the hidden homelessness of girls and women. "What happens to them? Where do they go? Try to get into the YWCA without any money or looking down at the heel. Charities take care of very few and only those that are called 'deserving.' The lone girl is under suspicion by the virgin women who dispense charity."[9] The "virgin women" Le Sueur mentions were, of course, Catholic nuns like the Sisters of Charity of Providence in Seattle. Hazel Wolf talked about the similarities between prostitutes and nuns: "They have a lot in common. At one time, nuns were considered the leftovers of society, the rejects. . . . Prostitution was another alternative to marriage. The prostitutes came from orphanages or poverty-stricken, miserable home lives. It was a very, very hard way to earn a living and prostitutes didn't live long."[10] She added that she loved both the nuns and the prostitutes from her childhood; the prostitutes she knew wanted out of "the life" but had no other viable options.

When Wolf first moved to Seattle she essentially was homeless and "couch surfed," living with various friends in apartments and rooming houses. While staying at one of these places she successfully fought a sexual assault by the husband of one of her friends. She was awakened by him in her bed. He was attempting to rape her. She pushed him off, escaped, and walked the streets of downtown Seattle all night until she found another female friend to take her in. She never told the first friend what had happened. Reflecting on this event, Wolf maintained that she had done the right thing in not reporting the incident to anyone, explaining that men "have urges" after all and that it was important not to ruin their reputations. It appears that after this experience she chose to stay with women only, and that is how she ended up living at the women's shelter on Profanity Hill.

Profanity Hill got its name from several factors. The first, and the one most often repeated, is that when King County had its odd-looking cupolaed courthouse built at the top of Yesler Hill, lawyers cursed loudly while climbing the steep steps along Terrace Street from downtown. The wealthy "first families" of Seattle also built their lavish Victorian homes at the top of this hill, Seattle's "first" hill. They wanted to be close to downtown yet sufficiently above and away from the noise, smells, and riffraff, especially from the Skid Road area along the waterfront. "Uphill" became a common term meaning to be in a better, more rarefied place.[11]

Yesler Hill was Seattle's first "good neighborhood," and at that time it was exclusively white. But by the beginning of World War I, the wealthy families had all moved to outlying communities with explicitly racial restrictive covenants—such as north to Capitol Hill and to the Olmsted-designed gated community, the Highlands Commons. A housing covenant for Ravenna, an area adjacent to the newer location of the University of Washington, stated, "No person of any other than the White or Caucasian race shall use or occupy any building or lot, except that this covenant shall not prevent occupancy by domestic servants of a different race domiciled with an owner or tenant."[12]

Some Seattle area housing covenants barred ownership or rental to "Hebrews" (Jews), or to Muslims, or to "Asiatics." The Victorian mansions on Yesler Hill were turned into low-income hotels, rooming houses, and brothels. The buildings fell into disrepair. Small wooden shacks were built around them and cascaded down the hillside onto Skid Road. One of the few areas without racial covenants, Yesler Hill was one of Seattle's most diverse neighborhoods. The second reason for the name Profanity Hill was because this area became Seattle's largest and most visible shacktown, "an unrelieved slum smack against the police station, the city and county government buildings, and the financial section."[13]

John Olmsted, the nephew and adopted son of famed American landscape architect Frederick Law Olmsted, was hired by the Seattle City Council between 1903 and the beginning of World War I to develop Seattle's parks, greenspaces, boulevards, and new University of Washington campus, which became the site of the 1909 Alaska-Yukon-Pacific Exposition. He also designed gated, whites-only communities, such as the Highlands Commons. This was part of the national City Beautiful movement with its emphasis on a uniquely American urban-planning process to bring civic pride, health, tourists, and increased prosperity to city dwellers. When he first came to Seattle, Olmsted was horrified by the housing on Profanity Hill and Skid Road, calling the diversity of people mingling there "race suicide."[14]

Race suicide, an idea associated with the eugenics movement, referred to the belief that the white Anglo-Saxon and Protestant "race" was not reproducing fast enough, especially in comparison with the high birth rates of immigrant and Catholic people in the United States. President Theodore Roosevelt, besides derisively admonishing the country to discount "hyphenated Americans," was a proponent of the concept of race suicide. In a widely influential 1905 address he gave to the National Congress of Mothers, he blamed women—understood to be white Anglo-Saxon women—for race suicide. He specifically blamed the use of birth control measures like the diaphragm and women's increased pursuit of higher education, which he termed "a sterile pseudo-intellectuality," for decreasing the birth rates of "desirable" Americans. According to Roosevelt, "the first and greatest duty of [white] womanhood" was to bear and raise many healthy children.[15]

Ironically, the Catholic women's shelter on Profanity Hill where Wolf stayed did not accept women with children, but Wolf convinced the Sisters to let Nydia live with her at least part of the time. It is unclear how much Hazel Wolf had her daughter with her through much of Nydia's early years. Wolf was reticent to talk about this aspect of her life and about her two brief marriages. Her discomfort in talking about motherhood is understandable given the stigma associated with not being a full-time "good" mother, a stigma that continues today but was much worse back then. About her marriages, Wolf would only say that her husbands were decent men who did not abuse her, but she felt "trapped."

Nydia, writing later in life, stated that she was only with her mother about half of her childhood and was raised by her grand-mother, who had moved to Port Angeles, closer to Seattle than was Victoria. Wolf's mother lived in poverty and in her sixties rode the rails as a hobo with her son, traveling between Port Angeles and eastern Washington to visit relatives. Nydia wrote about her fractured schooling from moving around so much, spending time on her own in downtown Seattle, and being picked up by police and truant officers, who would return her to Wolf with admonishments for Wolf to find better housing.[16] This may partially explain Wolf's brief second marriage to an American logger from the Port Angeles area. On several occa-sions, Nydia bought ferry tickets to return to her grandmother in Port Angeles but was caught by police before she could leave Seattle. They returned her to Wolf.

■ ■ ■

Besides a paucity of safe, affordable housing for impoverished single mothers, there was a lack of affordable daycare for work-ing women in Seattle. Rev. Mark Matthews, even though he had opposed women's suffrage and remained conflicted about work-ing women in general and working mothers in particular, led an effort to open a childcare center and preschool for low-income working mothers at First Presbyterian Church.[17] The Seattle Day Nursery opened on Profanity Hill in 1909; it was the first such childcare institution in Washington State. It continues in opera-tion at its original location but has expanded across King County as the nonprofit childcare agency Childhaven.

In 1913, Washington became one of the first states in the na-tion to enact legislation to provide what was termed "mothers' pensions." This came about from a variety of forces, but the lead-ing one was likely the solidarity and strength of the women's groups that had brought women's suffrage to the state in 1910. They highlighted the feminization of poverty, although the over-representation of women in poverty due in large part to sexism would not be named that until the women's rights movement in the 1960s and 1970s. The early version of the mother's pension in Washington State stipulated a small stipend per child up to age fifteen to be paid to destitute women whose husbands were either dead, disabled, in prison, or in an insane asylum. Unmarried single women with children were excluded, as were mothers who were divorced or who were deemed by the courts to be "unfit" due to physical, mental, or "moral" defects. In 1919, the law was amended to include aid to unmarried and divorced women. The residency requirement was three years in the state and one year in the county where the woman applied for aid.[18]

There is no indication that Hazel Wolf ever applied for a mother's pension or took advantage of the little childcare available after she moved to Seattle and had Nydia living with her. Wolf obtained housing for herself and her daughter at the women's shelter on Profanity Hill and stayed there for eight years. Wolf worked a variety of low-paying, low-skilled jobs when she moved to Seattle, ranging from placing Made in Japan stickers on Easter bunnies, to waitressing at a downtown diner, to working as a secretary in an office. For obtaining jobs and housing, it helped considerably that Wolf was a white, English-speaking young woman born to a Protestant American mother. Wolf considered herself an atheist throughout her life, but she was baptized as an infant in a Victoria church by her Scottish grandmother, and she attended Catholic schools for at least part of her childhood. These factors likely helped her obtain and keep temporary housing at the women's shelter through St. Mark's Cathedral.

The Ku Klux Klan—the Second Klan as it is called now—was active in the Seattle area in the 1920s. Leaders and supporters of the Second Klan were virulent white supremacists, nativist and anti-Catholic.[19] In a Seattle-based Klan newspaper, the *Watcher on the Tower*, in 1922 H. H. Bower wrote a full-page statement, "Why I Am a Klansman," listing fourteen reasons. Number nine states, "Because the Ku Klux Klan is 100% for White Supremacy,

Restricted Immigration, Protestantism, and Americanism."[20] The largest nonwhite population in Seattle at that time were Japanese Americans, who mostly lived in the Skid Road area along Jackson Street and on Profanity Hill.

After their almost decade-long stay at the women's shelter on Profanity Hill, Wolf moved with Nydia to housing near the University of Washington north of downtown so that Nydia could attend one of the city's better high schools, Roosevelt. The room they rented did not have a shower or bath so they showered at the university gym. Wolf had completed her high school equivalency while in Seattle and began taking sociology and economics courses at the University of Washington with the plan to become a social worker. But Wolf became disillusioned with her university courses and with social work as a profession so she dropped out of college before obtaining her degree. She could not afford the rent for the room near the university so they moved to a less expensive rooming house closer to the women's shelter where they had lived.

President Franklin Delano Roosevelt had begun the Works Progress Administration (WPA) in May 1935 with the aim of putting people back to work and getting them off welfare and direct or indirect relief of any kind, which he believed demeaned and pauperized people. Wolf began working in a series of WPA jobs, including writing, acting, and helping to put on plays through the Federal Theatre Project (FTP).[21] With the FTP she helped produce educational plays like *Spirochete* about the unmentionable and untreatable disease syphilis, as well as *Power*, a popular play about the desirability of public ownership of utilities, such as electricity. *Spirochete* attempted to address the stigma and racism inherent in public perceptions of syphilis and other sexually transmitted infections. There was a widespread belief that syphilis was associated with poverty, prostitution, and racial minorities, especially Black people. *Power* had relevancy in a unique way since Seattle had the nation's first municipally owned hydroelectric project, City Light. But the play that Wolf talked about the most later in her life was *One-Third of a Nation*. She also referred to this play as "You Have to Have a Place to Live."[22]

Based on a speech by FDR about how one-third of the nation was living in substandard housing or in shacks and the linkages between poor housing and poor heath, *One-Third of a Nation* was developed in a summer workshop at Vassar College with the final script written by Arthur Arent in 1938. An example of a "living newspaper," each city's version of the play incorporated local newspaper headlines and statistics on housing, poverty, health, and social ills. It opened with a burning tenement building, which was followed by a scene in which a "founding father," the landlord of the tenement, stood on a patch of green grass. He held a sign stating, "This is mine / Keep off." The play concluded with a direct appeal to audience members to support low-income federal and local housing programs.[23]

Before the play opened, the Seattle-based FTP director, Esther Porter, spent time taking photographs of Seattle slums, including in Skid Road and on Profanity Hill, and trying to track down the landlords and owners of the land and buildings. She found so many linkages to prominent Seattle people and leading churches that this part of the play was suppressed. Instead, her photographs were displayed in the lobby of the theater, and a half dozen noncontroversial Seattle poverty, health, and housing statistics were sprinkled throughout the play, which remained set in New York City.[24]

Along with her WPA jobs, Wolf began working for the socialist Workers Alliance of Washington, Local No. 1, part of a national union of WPA workers, where she became head of the grievance committee. The Seattle branch of the Workers Alliance was at 94 Main Street, near the previous waterfront location of the Wayside Mission Hospital. Fittingly, the building currently is headquarters for the homelessness and poverty newspaper *Real Change*. "When someone needed help, I would lead a delegation down to the zone office and we'd fight for it," Wolf stated about her time there.[25] Wolf worked with men and women living in Skid Road and in Seattle's shacktowns, especially the nearby Hooverville, which had grown to more than 1,500 residents. Hooverville now had street signs, home addresses, a post office, an auxiliary police force, fire and sanitation workers, and elected leaders to work with city government officials. It even had a Hooverville college in the planning phase. Most Hooverville residents were men, but there were also women and more than a few children and teenagers.

Like the older hobo "jungles," or gathering places for homeless men on the outskirts of towns, Hooverville residents provided temporary shelter and even shared what food they had with railroad hobos and drifters passing through. It was common practice that when a Hooverville resident got a job and could move into a rooming house, he gifted his shack to someone who needed it. The residents of Hooverville preferred to live there instead of the temporary, crowded, and uncomfortable missions in Skid Road. Hooverville was racially integrated with unemployed homeless whites, Blacks, Asian Americans, and Native Americans living side by side. Another shacktown of more than a thousand people, Louisville, was located on Harbor Island. A considerable number of homeless people lived in the basements of abandoned buildings, and some slept on top of brick kilns at night to keep warm. In the words of historian Barron Lerner, "While other American cities had similar skid row populations, Seattle's Skid Road was distinctive, often representing the end of the line for migrants who had traveled west in search of work."[26]

Kicked out of his home in eastern Washington at age thirteen, Monte Holm was a railroad hobo for six years during the Depression before establishing a junk business north of Seattle. In his autobiography, Holm remembers his stay in the Seattle shacktown: "Hooverville resembled a small city of makeshift shelters with at least 1,000 people living there. . . . We found that some of the little shacks were for sale for as little as $10, but the person selling really didn't own the shack or property it was on. Still people had been there for years and it was a permanent home as far as they were concerned."[27]

Wolf was part of the effort in October 1938 to petition the Seattle City Council to stop evictions of residents of Hooverville. Signed by Vance Ardeune of the Workers Alliance, Local No. 1, the letter begins, "A critical situation has arisen in Hooverville wherein unemployed and aged people with no source of income are being evicted." He adds that the evictions "greatly affect the health and welfare of all the people of the city" and asks that the mayor and the city council "use police powers to stop homeless people from being evicted in face of a housing shortage and in face of the coming winter."[28]

■ ■ ■

The city council was receiving an increasing number of letters and petitions, mainly from people working in real estate and women's groups, demanding that the city address the "shacktown problem." In their view, the shacks and the residents of them were causing unsanitary and unsightly conditions for everyone, as well as reducing the property values of homeowners—and, by extension, reducing city revenue from property taxes. Shacktowns, also called shantytowns, were present in many urban areas throughout the United States. They were reminders of the poverty that had not been eliminated by the frontier expansion, and in the western states, they recalled much earlier "concerns over the uncivilized, 'savage' influence of the frontier."[29]

A *Seattle Post-Intelligencer* article from December 6, 1938, "Shacktown Boom Arouses Citizens," was accompanied by a striking photograph. Above the caption "Unwanted view: She gets a 'good' look at unsightly shanties," a Beacon Hill housewife identified as Mrs. John Redmond points out of her living room window at a shacktown below, which blends in with Hooverville on the former tidal flats. Besides the "unwanted view" of the "unsightly shacktowns" full of "swarming colonies of squatters," homeowners complain of men from the shacktown rummaging through their garbage cans late at night and the "constant begging at the doors for food or work." Another housewife interviewed for the article "thinks a number of Seattle's own poor are living in Shacktown but . . . a serious number of transients" are landing in Seattle and settling in the shanties. The reporter maintains that "none of those interviewed said they were in favor of driving the residents out of Shacktown without providing them with other homes." But she adds that they "condemned the policy that allowed the districts to spring up in the first place."[30]

The Seattle parks designed by Olmsted, which included Green Lake in North Seattle, became contentious areas due to the increasing number of homeless car and tent campers living there. Not only the Great Depression but also the effects of the Dust Bowl had driven entire families into cities like Seattle. Called "rubber hobos," they essentially were evacuees from a man-made (not a natural) environmental and economic disaster. In an echo of earlier back-to-the-land solutions to the growing homeless problem in US urban areas, there was a national back-to-the-farm campaign. There were rubber hobos and shacktown communities all over Seattle and King County, although the shacktowns were concentrated in low-lying areas around city garbage dumps and on undesirable land.[31]

A letter written to the Seattle City Council by May Gamble Young, who was representing the North End Progressive Club, a "society" whites-only women's group, complained of the "little colony of poverty stricken people who have built shacks in the sand at Interbay waterfront." This shacktown, built beside another city dump, had been dubbed "Jungle City." She invoked the "stranger" and wandering pauper aspect of the old Poor Laws by stating, "We recognize the fact that these people have drifted in from other parts of the country." This was a common—and largely false—assumption since studies showed that the overwhelming majority of shacktown residents were longtime residents of Washington State and of Seattle. Young concluded her letter by acknowledging "that it is unlawful to shoot or drown them. But—we want you to do *something* about it."[32]

The Seattle City Council responded to citizen complaints about the shantytowns by establishing the Shack Elimination Committee. This committee, formed in 1941, was headed by the commissioner of health and included the superintendent of buildings, the chief of police, and the chief of the fire department.[33] They first commissioned a study of the "shack problem."[34] Seattle officials had begun to be alarmed at the possibility of the residents of Hooverville and other Seattle shantytowns filing for squatters' rights—and in the case of Hooverville at least, city officials had begun to view the land the squatters lived on as valuable property.[35] Hooverville, built on the former Skinner and Eddy Shipyard, was on land now owned by the Port of Seattle, which planned to develop the area. And Seattle, as well as the entire nation, was mobilizing to enter World War II. Hooverville residents were ordered to leave their homes, and the shacktown was razed in April 1941.[36] Some of the former residents of shacktowns obtained jobs and could move into better housing. But many others simply moved to more marginalized areas, such as along the Duwamish River.[37]

■ ■ ■

One Friday in the late 1930s when Hazel Wolf went to the zone office for her weekly food voucher, a social worker noticed on her records that Wolf had completed thirty-two credits of sociology courses and asked her to apply for a job there as a social worker. "Well, I am a social worker," Wolf reported that she replied. "I am doing exactly that. The only difference between you and me is that I can do and say as I please, but you are tied to all these rules and regulations in that manual."[38] Wolf added that social workers were, for the most part, compassionate women, but they "were buffers, 'interpreting the policy of the administration.' That was the jargon they used."

Social work, along with public health nursing, had grown out of the earlier "friendly visitors" approach to charity work by religious and secular entities. As such, both were overwhelmingly female-dominated vocations. In social work's drive to become more of a profession in the United States, beginning in 1921 with the establishment of the American Association of Social Workers, social workers claimed individual client or family casework as their special area of expertise.[39] Thus, they formed medical social work, school-based social work, and psychiatric social work, all using the individual casework model as the basis.[40] This individual focus aligned with the prevailing American belief that an individual's faults were the cause of poverty and ill health. To back this up and to create a "science" of social work, the expanding field of sociology stepped in.

Social workers and university-based sociologists had begun to fill bookshelves with numerous studies, such as Alice Willard Solenberger's *One Thousand Homeless Men: A Study of Original Records* and Nels Anderson's *The Hobo: The Sociology of the Homeless Man*.[41] Significantly, both of these researchers, but especially Solenberger, emphasized social disconnection, like broken family ties, and deemphasized the lack of housing in their descriptions and definitions of homeless men.

In Seattle, these types of studies included the 1930 *Facilities for Housing, Medical Care, and Other Services for Homeless Men in Seattle 1929–30* by Allen Potter and a 1935 thesis by University of Washington student Donald Francis Roy.[42] For a term paper, sociology student Annette de Vol Trumbull completed an oral history in 1935 with the unofficial mayor of Hooverville.[43] These research studies began to "scientifically" and allegedly objectively sort homeless people into categories. For instance, Solenberger in *One Thousand Homeless Men* used categories such as "crippled and maimed," "insane, feeble-minded, and epileptic," "homeless old men," "confirmed wanderers or 'tramps,'" and "homeless, vagrant, and runaway boys." Nels Anderson added to these the category of "sexual perversion" with a frank discussion of widespread same-sex practices, especially adult railroad hobos preying on homeless teenage boys. These studies were attempts to document the problem in order to develop and test scientific solutions to poverty and homelessness. Anderson, who was homeless and a railroad hobo as a teenager, including in Washington State, wrote a sequel and parody of his own book *The Hobo* later in his life. Using the pen name Dean Stiff in *The Milk and Honey Route: A Handbook for Hobos*, Anderson wrote, "Social workers are a recent development of the machine age. They are the ambulance corps of the capitalist system and as such they have one objective in all that they do." The objective of social workers, in his view, was to make people work.[44]

Progressive Era reformers, such as public health nurse and settlement house leader in New York City Lillian Wald, had pushed for systemic societal changes to address inadequate housing and poverty and not only provide health education for poor people.[45] She and other women reformers called for the establishment of district (community-based) nursing modeled on the system established in England by Florence Nightingale. Although not successful in instituting district nursing, their work led to the establishment of the federal Children's Bureau to address infant mortality, child labor, childhood immunization, and other related issues.

The rise of the power of organized groups of physicians, which were essentially trade unions, including the American Medical Association, at first allowed this since the women public health nurses and midwives focused on preventative health measures and the physicians focused on the more lucrative curative medicine. The public health nurses and midwives had to promise to refer medical cases to physicians, thus guaranteeing physician sovereignty in medical care. When physicians began to specialize in pediatrics and obstetrics and realized the revenue they could make in preventative, well-woman, and well-baby care, they effectively undermined the work of midwives and public health nurses.[46] Around the time of World War I, Lillian Wald also advocated for women's suffrage, racial justice, women's trade unions, and anti-militarism. For these efforts, Wald and other Progressive reformers were labeled un-American and were caught up in the first red scare at the end of World War I. This effectively undermined their reform efforts.[47]

As part of Roosevelt's New Deal, the National Health Act of 1939 was introduced to strengthen national public health efforts, including fighting high rates of syphilis and tuberculosis, and to expand healthcare access to all Americans. Not surprisingly, the American Medical Association and the pharmaceutical industry vehemently opposed this effort and labeled it "socialized medicine."[48] This original act was blocked, only to be repackaged and reintroduced as the 1945 Social Security expansion bill under President Harry S. Truman. But the second red scare and the rise of McCarthyism in the United States gave even more strength to the loud claims by the American Medical Association of it being socialized medicine, and it was again defeated.

■ ■ ■

Hazel Wolf was in the welfare line at the zone office one day in 1935 when she picked up a flyer with information about a petition to the state legislature for unemployment insurance. This led her to a Communist Party meeting, but the police were evicting the person holding the meeting. She assisted with putting back the person's belongings, which had been dumped on the sidewalk by police. Seattle police routinely harassed known and suspected communists throughout the 1920s and 1930s, including after 1933 through evictions and deportations, using the increased power of the US Immigration and Naturalization Service (INS).[49] The police also arrested and charged suspected communists using the old vagrancy laws.

The Depression era communist and homeless author Tillie Olsen describes this in her autobiographical "Thousand Dollar Vagrant."[50] She tells of being arrested in San Francisco during the 1934 West Coast waterfront strike. Since it was not illegal to be a communist, she was charged with vagrancy and fined $1,000 because she refused to tell police her real name or her address. People associated with the Communist Party were arrested and deported by the INS if their US citizenship was in question, or they were charged with vagrancy, mainly because, like Olsen, people refused to give their real names and addresses in order to protect their friends and families from similar harassment. Olsen writes, "And even if you do show your 'visible means of support'—you're still a vagrant."

Of her involvement with the Communist Party in Seattle, Wolf emphasized that they did direct action, they helped fight evictions, and they provided food, firewood, and other necessities to impoverished people. The Communist Party and the socialist Workers Alliance were community- and neighborhood-based. This appealed to Wolf given her connections to her impoverished childhood shacktown community and her growing connections with Seattle communities marginalized by poverty, race, and homelessness. Commenting on why she joined the Communist Party, Wolf said that it helped her not feel so alone and helpless, plus "it was necessary because of the suffering people endured."[51] Although the Communist Party in the United States was rigidly patriarchal, the "homegrown" version in the Pacific Northwest allowed room for women to step into leadership positions. For a while, Wolf was the head of the Communist Party's office in the majority Black Central District just northeast of Profanity Hill. In addition, she assisted with the formation and running of the Washington State Pension Union, which was one of the first state old age pensions in the country and preceded the establishment of the federal Social Security Act of 1935.

These factors led to the US postmaster general under FDR, James A. Farley, referring in a speech to "the forty-seven states in the Union and the soviet of Washington."[52] Commenting on these same factors, the Seattle-born but by then "highbrow" East Coast author Mary McCarthy wrote, "The state of Washington is in ferment; it is wild, comic, theatrical, dishonest, disorganized, hopeful; but it is not revolutionary."[53] Washington State and Seattle may not have been revolutionary, but they were uniquely left-leaning. The Washington Communist Party, while "never a broad-based mass organization . . . may have achieved a greater degree of influence, and therefore, success than was the case in other parts of the United States."[54]

■ ■ ■

Rev. Mark Matthews of First Presbyterian Church, who saw himself as a moral compass for Seattle, was a staunch prohibitionist, and as early as 1905 he advocated for Seattle to go dry. He acknowledged the social community-gathering function of saloons and advocated for them to be replaced with coffeehouses "not intended as a hoboes' resort nor a pauperizing institution." He saw the coffeehouse as a sort of community center where people could read newspapers, magazines, and literature, look for jobs, and write letters to their mothers telling of their whereabouts— an acknowledgment of the large number of single transient men in Seattle.[55] Although the coffee-house model would not take off for another sixty or so years, prohibition did. On January 1, 1916, the state of Washington went dry, and Seattle became the largest dry city in the world. In 1920 the Volstead Act—enforcing the Eighteenth Amendment—went into effect.[56] The National Prohibition Act brought prohibition to the entire United States. Locally and nationally, prohibition efforts were led by women's temperance groups, which focused on the linkage between alcohol, intimate partner violence, and the impoverishment of women and children caused by men's drinking.

■ ■ ■

Early in the twentieth century, Seattle was statistically the healthiest city in the nation.[57] Residents of the city and King County, however, had higher than average rates of suicide and tuberculosis—both with the highest concentration among residents of the Skid Road area. Suicide by hanging and from "illuminating gas" were most common for middle-aged and older single men living in cheap rooming houses in Skid Road. A report linked this high suicide rate to loneliness and disconnection among the men.[58]

Tuberculosis—called the "white plague" for the pallor of TB patients—was Seattle's leading cause of death and was linked with poverty, homelessness, overcrowded living conditions, alcoholism, and poor nutrition. By this time, the cause of tuberculosis was known, but the cure for it was elusive. Antibiotics to treat TB had not been discovered, so the main treatments consisted of rest, preferably in clean, cool outside air, and in extreme cases, surgical removal of infected lung tissue.[59] Since TB was considered a social disease akin to venereal disease, Washington State passed a law in 1909 banning marriage for people with tuberculosis—and mental illness, feeble-mindedness, epilepsy, and venereal diseases.

Also in 1909, Washington became the second state in the nation after Indiana to pass eugenics laws for the forced sterilization of anyone accused of "carnal abuse of a female person under 10 years of age, or rape, or an habitual criminal."[60] Oregon physician and temperance worker Bethenia Owens-Adair and other Progressive Era women and physicians advocated for these eugenics laws. Then, in 1921, the eugenics laws in the state mandated that the superintendents of state mental hospitals, including Western State Hospital, and custodial schools report "all feebleminded, insane, epileptic, habitual criminals, moral degenerates, and sexual perverts" capable of reproduction who "would probably become a social menace or wards of the state." The law allowed and even recommended the forced sterilization of such people. "Sexual perverts" included, of course, LGBTQ people, as well as prostitutes.[61]

Between 1921 and 1942, when it was outlawed, there were a total of 685 involuntary sterilizations in Washington State. Of these, 501 (73 percent) were women. There are indications that among the women involuntarily sterilized, a disproportionate number were women of color and especially African American women since deeply entrenched racism portrayed Black women as hypersexual. LGBTQ people of all genders were overrepresented as well in these forced sterilizations.[62] Beginning soon after statehood, Washington had sodomy laws outlawing "crimes against nature," effectively outlawing homosexuality. These laws remained in effect until 1975. The LGBTQ population was discriminated against in all aspects of life, including jobs, healthcare, and housing.

Beginning in the early part of the twentieth century, Seattle reformers called for the city and county to address the health needs and issues of the considerable and growing homeless and indigent population. Rev. Matthews advocated for free medical care for homeless and indigent patients and for the University of Washington to open a medical school through which medical students could provide free care. This was not done until 1946, but the University of Washington did open the first official school of nursing in the West in 1923; it was also only the second university-affiliated school of nursing in the country. Unfortunately, the tuberculosis public health nurse who founded the school, Elizabeth Sterling Soule, was overtly racist and refused to admit Black nursing students. The school of nursing was part of the new Harborview Hospital from its beginning, with a separate Nurses Hall adjacent to the hospital to house the nurses and students who worked there. Harborview hired Seattle's first Black nurse in 1943, and the University of Washington finally graduated its first Black nurse in 1949.

Rev. Matthews called for a city hospital—which Seattle opened in 1909 in the city-county building—to take over the patients from the Wayside Emergency Hospital, which had been started by Alexander de Soto. King County maintained its hospital at the old poor farm location in Georgetown and in 1909 added a new brick hospital there that had a 225-patient capacity. King County added tents along the Duwamish River as open-air places to treat tuberculosis patients.[63] The city of Seattle, besides operating the city hospital, opened its own TB facility, Firland Sanatorium, in the northern part of town. During this time, it was common practice for doctors to send Native Alaskan people—including young children—to Seattle for treatment of TB in sanatoriums such as Firland. As Coll Thrush points out, this further fractured families and contributed to the high rates of homelessness among Native Americans.[64]

In the early 1940s, Wolf was diagnosed with TB and began a nine-month-long treatment at Firland. She reported that she had been feeling unwell for some time before finally being diagnosed. It is likely that she first contracted tuberculosis either as a child living in the shacktown in Victoria or in the crowded women's shelter in Seattle on Profanity Hill. In characteristic form, Wolf claimed to have cured herself with humor, playing pranks on the nurses and other patients. Once she was discharged, she returned to Firland to visit patients she had befriended. She enjoyed telling of the time she smuggled a goldfish in a bowl into the facility for a patient who missed being in nature and having pets. The nurses confiscated the fish, and the patient died soon after.[65]

. . .

"Above the Brightness of the Sun: Service." This is the statement on a promotional brochure for the opening of Harborview Hospital in 1931. The saying is accompanied by a drawing of the grand art deco hospital on Profanity Hill, the rising sun above it, and above the sun, a young nurse tending to a young man with a bandaged head who is lying in a hospital bed. The brochure's image reflected the fact that many people in Seattle believed that Harborview Hospital's mission came from heaven even though it was a secular institution.[66] Harborview Hospital exemplified not only service but also the power of the science of medicine. The hospital was outfitted with the newest medical and surgical equipment and would soon become a national and even international leader in emergency and burn care.

Harborview Hospital was originally called King County Hospital Number One to differentiate it from the former King County Hospital in Georgetown, which served aged and convalescing patients. The Georgetown facility was designated as King County Hospital Number Two and remained there until airplane noise and air pollution from the nearby Boeing Field forced its closure in the 1950s. Harborview was the direct result of the findings of a medical consultant's report in 1927. The report had noted the inadequate and unsafe patient and employee conditions in the various city and county healthcare facilities.[67] At the Detention Hospital and Venereal Clinic on top of Profanity Hill in the old King County Court House, the consultant found deplorable conditions; for example, windows in the women's "prostitution" venereal disease ward were nailed shut because women had died trying to escape. Based on this report, Seattle closed its hospital along Yesler Way and transferred patients to the new Harborview Hospital.

If that bandaged patient in the hospital pamphlet's illustration had been well enough to be taken in a wheelchair one late winter afternoon in 1932 to a southwest-facing glass atrium high up in the hospital, he would have gazed out at the new Seattle Marine Hospital on the top of Beacon Hill. Between the two hospitals, he would have seen the "unrelieved slum" of the shacktown cascading down Profanity Hill and blending into Skid Road and Hooverville below. People in Seattle had "fled to outlying streetcar suburbs and away from the waterfront and downtown hillsides synonymous with disorder and disease. . . . Many urbanites continued to associate poor health with poor landscapes and poor people, crystallizing fears over urban decay."[68]

■ ■ ■

In 1939, Jesse Epstein, a recent University of Washington law school graduate, was hired to head the newly formed Seattle Housing Authority to address the city's poor housing conditions. One of his first tasks was to conduct a study of housing in Seattle. This WPA-funded survey of Seattle housing in 1939–1940 found 28.5 percent of the 124,774 dwelling units to be substandard, one of the highest percentages of substandard housing in the nation's urban areas. The housing inventory included 1,687 "shacks" and 950 houseboats, called "shackboats," along the shores of the Duwamish River, Lake Washington, and Lake Union.[69]

From the beginning, Epstein had as his priority getting rid of the "slum" on Profanity Hill. Epstein made connections in his numerous public speeches between the impoverished residents of this shacktown area and the high costs to the city and county for healthcare, police, and fire services. He made reference to the shacktown being a direct pipeline of indigent patients into the adjacent Harborview Hospital. Epstein positioned the Seattle Housing Authority to take advantage of new federal public housing funding in order to clear this shacktown and build a forty-three-acre public housing project, Yesler Terrace.

To provide better housing in urban areas, to clear slums, and to revive the construction industry, the US Congress passed the National Housing Act (the Wagner-Steagall Act) in September 1937, establishing the US Housing Authority, the first national housing program. Although intended mainly to provide public housing for middle- and working-class white families, efforts by more liberal-minded people at the federal level established the "neighborhood composition rule." This allowed for racially integrated public housing in areas that had already integrated.[70] Since Profanity Hill in Seattle was a racially mixed area, Epstein developed Yesler Terrace to match this. When it opened in 1941, Yesler Terrace became the nation's first racially integrated public housing.

A possible classmate of Hazel Wolf when she was at the University of Washington was the social worker Irene Burns Miller. In 1940, Miller was a widow with a young daughter to support so she took a job as a social worker with the Seattle Housing Authority. Jesse Epstein hired her to "clear out" and relocate the more than a thousand residents of the Profanity Hill "slum" area to make way for the new Yesler Terrace public housing project.

In her memoir *Profanity Hill*, Miller writes about the racism she encountered when she tried to assist a widowed Black woman and her children to find an apartment near the University of Washington, where the woman was a student.[71] Landlords made it clear that they were willing to rent apartments to Miller, who was white, but not to the Black student. She also writes about "society women" asking her if she was afraid of being raped by Black men in the area. Miller reveals that there were hidden race and welfare quotas, with only a certain percentage of "acceptable" Black people and welfare recipients allowed to move into the new housing. Yesler Terrace was exclusively for families with US citizenship, so many of the single, unmarried, and possibly not heterosexual people who had lived there before were not eligible to return. In the end, Yesler Terrace was helpful to many working-class, mainly white families, but did not address the housing needs of the poor and homeless.

■ ■ ■

Wolf had neglected to apply for US citizenship when she relocated to Seattle. This fact, combined with her history of membership and activity in the Communist Party, led to her arrest in 1949 by the INS for being a subversive alien. This began her fifteen-year fight with the INS, which tried to deport her to either Canada or the United Kingdom, even though she had been born to an American mother and her second marriage was to an American. During this time, she worked as a legal secretary for Seattle civil rights lawyer John Caughlan, who helped her fight deportation. Wolf finally gained US citizenship in 1974 and retired on Social Security income and a Seattle Housing Authority rental subsidy for an apartment on Capitol Hill.[72]

But Hazel Wolf never really retired. She began working as a volunteer with various environmental groups, including the Audubon Society, where her left-leaning politics irritated many society women. She extended her work to include environmental justice issues, calling attention to the high rates of cancer and childhood asthma for people—mainly Native Americans and other people of color—along the Duwamish River in Georgetown near where the King County Poor Farm had been.[73] She asked pointed questions, such as "Are there abandoned landfills bearing toxics located in low-income Georgetown and none in affluent Laurelhurst?"[74]

As she approached her hundredth birthday, she was on the board of directors for the Country Doctor Clinic, a community health clinic located near her apartment on Capitol Hill. She received her healthcare there, or at least what little she needed since she remained in robust health. Her care mostly consisted of preventative treatment, such as immunizations and having her ears cleaned and her toenails clipped. She described a homeless mentally ill man at the clinic and others of the "great unwashed" as "her people" and saw their connection with the people she had grown up with in the shacktown of her childhood. She died at 101, peacefully in her sleep, soon after asking a healthcare worker for a cookie.

6

THRESHOLD

Never mind the body lying inert in the doorway. The body is
there to remind you of those who went before, of those who tried
to find their way out, their way home.
—Josephine Ensign, *Soul Stories: Voices from the Margins*

In the late afternoon of a warm April day in 1983 on First Avenue at Pike Place Market in Seattle, near where Princess Angeline's shack had stood, a thin, petite, white teenage girl dressed
in a cropped T-shirt and high-waisted jeans stood on the sidewalk. Smoking, talking, and laughing with two other teen girls,
her shag-cut brown hair bounced as she laughed and glanced
at passing cars. Michael Jackson music from a boom box competed with hymns sung by an evangelist on the street corner.
A man in a three-piece, navy, pin-striped suit walked by and
turned to look at the girls' backsides. Graffiti on a wall nearby
included "Rat," "Mike," "Dope Head," "Tramp," and "Stephen B.
Was Here." Smells from the fish market mixed with stale frying
oil from a burger shop. The shop window displayed prominent
No Loitering signs. Loudly squawking seagulls circled overhead
and fought over trash in overflowing dumpsters. The insistent

staccato clanging of a railroad crossing signal drifted uphill, accompanied by the low horns of ferryboats.

A middle-aged woman with long, curly, black hair and a zoom-lensed camera stood nearby taking photographs of street scenes and the teenagers. A Seattle police cruiser driven by a blond-moustached officer rolled through just as the shag-haircut girl slipped into the front passenger seat of a baby blue Oldsmobile Cutlass driven by an older white man. Both the photographer and the police officer watched as the man drove away with the girl, who briefly turned and waved at her friends. Perhaps the man driving the Oldsmobile was her grandfather or her father. And perhaps he was not.

Thirteen-year-old Erin Blackwell, whose street name was "Tiny," had school photographs from grades 1–5 among her belongings stored at her mother's downtown studio apartment. The apartment was above a tavern, which was where her mother, Pat, spent most of her evenings, drinking. Pat, who worked as a waitress at a diner, had a series of live-in boyfriends who also drank and physically abused her. It is unclear what, if anything, these men might have done to the young Erin. An only child, Erin did not know who her father was, and her mother refused to tell her, with the rationale being that she did not like the man. Freckle-faced, apple-cheeked Erin smiles broadly in all five Seattle public school photographs. In her third-grade photograph, she is wearing a Brownie uniform. In the picture from fourth grade, she is wearing a T-shirt with the band Kiss on the front. In fifth grade, she has the beginning of a shag haircut and is wearing a pink plaid western shirt. She added sparkly stickers of a unicorn on the upper corners of this photograph. It was her last school photograph. And it appears to be the last image of her without permanent scars on her face.

The black-haired woman taking photographs that day of Pike Place Market street scenes and of Erin Blackwell was forty-three-year-old Mary Ellen Mark. Mark, a New York City photojournalist by then well known for her sympathetic portrayals of poverty, homelessness, madness, and disabilities, was on assignment for *Life* magazine. The assignment was to document the growing national problem of runaway and street-involved teens. Accompanied by the tenacious journalist Cheryl McCall, Mark chose Seattle because it was then considered to be one of America's most livable cities. If runaways and street youth were found in Seattle, then they could be anywhere. In their July 1983 *Life* magazine article, "Streets of the Lost," Mark and McCall documented the seedy underbelly of Seattle and a different truth about its livability—that livability was increasing for some people but for others, life in Seattle was barely survivable.[1] Erin Blackwell—Tiny—as a runaway teen in Seattle became Mary Ellen Mark's artistic muse and the subject of her most famous photograph.

■ ■ ■

Pike Place Market, Seattle's first sanitary and direct-to-the-public farmers market, with its large red neon sign and clock and rambling arcades overlooking Puget Sound, had survived the wrecking balls of developers in the 1960s and 1970s who wanted to build upscale skyscrapers on the increasingly valuable land.[2] A Seattle architect, University of Washington professor, and activist, Victor Steinbrueck, who had filled sketchbooks with Hooverville shacks during the Great Depression, helped form the group Friends of the Market. They successfully fought off developers and worked to secure the designation of the area as a historic district. Steinbrueck also helped Seattle boosters to designate the original Skid Road south of Yesler Way as the Pioneer Square Historic District in 1970.

Pioneer Square became one of the nation's first federally designated national historic districts as a link to the US frontier past. In both Pioneer Square and Pike Place Market, provision for low-income, subsidized housing was built into the development plans. Some of this focus on the inclusion of low-income housing was motivated by a social consciousness and some of it by pragmatic entrepreneurial interests. For instance, Bill Speidel, one of the leaders of the movement to create the Pioneer Square Historic District and founder of the lucrative Seattle Underground Tour, joked that if the Skid Road "homeless bums" were cleared out of the area, he would have to hire actors to replace them to maintain an authentically gritty, frontier-worthy Seattle urban scene.[3]

In the 1960s Seattle also reflected the country's New Frontier, President John F. Kennedy's focus on the space race, and the rise of science and technology as a cure for all of society's ills, including poverty. In his 1960 acceptance speech as the Democratic nominee at the Los Angeles convention, Kennedy evoked the old frontier of the American West and "the pioneers of old. . . . their motto was not 'every man for himself' but 'all for the common cause.'" He then alluded to Frederick Jackson Turner's 1893 closing of the frontier. Kennedy countered this with a vision of the New Frontier, which would address "the uncharted areas of science and space, unsolved problems of peace and war, unconquered pockets of ignorance and prejudice, unanswered questions of poverty and surplus." He asked listeners "to be pioneers on that new frontier."[4] Seattle's 1962 world's fair, the Century 21 Exposition, featured a space theme, an elevated monorail, and the towering Space Needle, as well as a popular adults-only area on Show Street, "Peep Backstage U.S.A.," and a show featuring naked "girls of the galaxy."[5]

In mid-November 1961, President Kennedy visited Seattle and stayed downtown at the Olympic Hotel (now the Fairmont Hotel), the building site of the first Territorial University. He gave a speech at the University of Washington on the Cold War with Russia and invoked the pre–Civil War "dark days of 1861 when this great University was founded." He added, "This territory had only the simplest elements of civilization. And this city had barely begun to function. But a university was one of their earliest thoughts—and they summed it up in the motto they adopted [for the University of Washington]: 'Let There Be Light.'"[6]

Kennedy did not mention in his speech that the university's unofficial motto should have been "Let there be white girls and women." Or more specifically, "Let there be white, Protestant, educated girls and women," given the mission of Asa Mercer, the first president of the Territorial University of Washington. Beginning in 1864, when the Civil War had created young widowed women and a dearth of eligible bachelors while the fledgling Seattle had a surplus of bachelors and very few woman, Mercer established a business scheme to import girls and women. As Murray Morgan states, "The idea had an understandable appeal to the twenty-two-year-old university president, who was unmarried and moral."[7] Unmarried, yes, but whether he was moral is questionable. Mercer only wanted to import "proper," educated, white, and Protestant young women, so he recruited from the mill town of Lowell, Massachusetts—not far from Ashburnham, where Seattle's first homeless person, Edward Moore, had hung himself and was now buried.

What is not well known in the story of the "Mercer Girls" is that Asa Mercer ended up kidnapping at least some of the young women as he sailed with them to Seattle: he would not allow them to stay in Chile, where they had met dashing young Chilean soldiers.[8] This was a form of human and sex trafficking although the federal and territorial laws of the time did not regulate this sort of activity.[9] Mercer eventually married one of the young women he had "imported." In the fall of 1968, ABC-TV debuted a new comedy western series, *Here Come the Brides*. Early scripts of this series featured a feisty Seattle brothel keeper named Momma Damnation in a nod to the real-life Madame Damnable. But the Momma Damnation character was taken out of the series because she was deemed too racy for a family TV show.[10] *Here Come the Brides* ran for two seasons and was popular in the Seattle area.

More recently, it has become known that an unnamed King County sheriff supplied President Kennedy with two female prostitutes during his 1961 visit to Seattle. As the sheriff dropped off the two young women at Kennedy's Olympic Hotel suite, the sheriff was overheard by Secret Service agent Larry Newman admonishing the women that if they ever told anyone about this sexual liaison he would make sure they both went to Steilacoom—Western State Hospital—and he would ensure that they would never get out.[11] Since Kennedy's sexual proclivities are well known by now, this episode reveals more about the scope of Seattle and King County police corruption and the abuse of girls and women in prostitution. It emphasizes the normalizing of prostitution and gender-based violence, as well as Washington State's long legacy of eugenics laws extending to prostitutes, who were deemed to be "sexual perverts" in need of being locked in insane asylums and sterilized.

■ ■ ■

With a local economy reliant no longer on timber but rather on the aerospace company Boeing, the Seattle area had expanded during and after World War II. Many families lived in modest houses built in Seattle's growing and largely white suburbs. Single men and women—disproportionately Native American and other people of color—who were living closer to poverty and homelessness, lived in the still abundant, yet decaying single room occupancy (SRO) hotels downtown. These SROs were concentrated in what became Pioneer Square, north along the waterfront to Pike Place Market, and into Belltown. With business pressures to revitalize downtown Seattle, along with tighter fire safety standards following deadly fires in the wood-frame SRO hotels, by the early 1980s more than three-quarters of the SRO low-income housing stock had been lost.[12]

The post–World War II national emphasis on the growth of highways and interstates affected Seattle, especially with the

1962 completion of I-5 through the center of the city. The building of this highway wiped out a large section of Yesler Terrace, destroying 263 low-income units of public housing which, at the time, were only twenty years old. Interstate 5 created a large gash, effectively dividing the city, and created significant noise and air pollution, which continues today.

The aptly named Empire Expressway, slated to cut through the heart of the Central District, was effectively blocked by a coalition of Seattle activists that included the Black Panthers, environmental groups, and the League of Women Voters. The Empire Expressway was slated to run through Georgetown, near where the King County Poor Farm and Hospital had stood, up through the Central District—then designated as a slum in need of clearance—through the University of Washington Arboretum, and up to Bothell at the north end of Lake Washington. It was later renamed the R. H. Thompson Expressway for the ambitious Seattle engineer of the early 1900s who washed away parts of Seattle's hills, including First Hill. One of the main purposes of this expressway was to clear the inner-city, mainly African American slum of the Central District and make it easier for white flight to the suburbs. Parts of the expressway were built before the project was permanently blocked. Dubbed the "bridges to nowhere," these sections provided diving platforms into Lake Washington for generations of University of Washington students, as well as shelter for homeless people for half a century, before being torn down beginning in 2018.[13]

Following Kennedy's assassination in November 1963, President Lyndon B. Johnson began the War on Poverty as part of his Great Society vision. In the flurry of resulting federal legislation addressing national poverty rates, the Demonstration Cities and Metropolitan Development Act of 1966 began what was known as the Model Cities program to address urban high-poverty areas, or slums.[14] Seattle's boosters and politicians billed the city as a young, innovative place with "relatively new slums" that had not reached "the final stages of decay" or the urban blight of older cities.[15] They designated the original Skid Road area of Pioneer Square, parts of the waterfront along First Avenue, First Hill, and the Central District as the slum area to be revitalized. Seattle became the nation's first recipient of Model Cities funding and created a five-year plan to revitalize its slum areas.[16] A 1971 evaluation report of the Seattle Model Cities program highlights continuing racial discrimination in selling or renting housing, a net loss of close to 500 single-family homes, and public housing agencies reporting wait times of four months for housing projects and two years for leased housing. The report states that there was a well-founded desire for the Seattle Model Cities program to "maintain a 'low profile' in order not to excite undue expectations in the community."[17]

■ ■ ■

By the time Erin Blackwell was born in May 1969, Seattle was slipping into yet another deep recession, playing out the boom-and-bust cycle that has characterized the city from its earliest days. Between 1968 and 1971, Boeing laid off 86,000 people due to the national recession. This became known as the Boeing Bust. Washington State unemployment hit 14 percent, the highest in the nation.[18] In April 1971, two Seattle area real estate agents put up a billboard on Route 99, Pacific Highway South, near the Sea-Tac Airport. The sign showed a bare lightbulb and read "Will the Last Person Leaving Seattle—Turn Out the Lights."[19] For the first time in the city's history, except perhaps right after the short-lived Battle of Seattle in 1856, Seattle experienced a net loss in population.

Erin Blackwell's mother, who worked as a waitress in downtown diners, likely was hit hard by this recession, and its effects could have worsened her growing alcohol dependency, as well as housing instability for her and Erin. Harking back to the years of the Great Depression, food banks, housing support, and suicide prevention efforts proliferated in and around Seattle. So many people threw themselves off the observation deck at the top of the Space Needle that it was enclosed. Soon after assuming office in 1969, President Richard M. Nixon declared the War on Drugs, calling illegal drugs "public enemy number one." A University of Washington psychology student, Ted Bundy, worked on the hotline for the Seattle Crisis Clinic, which included a special youth hotline. During the same period, Bundy was brutally raping and murdering female students from the University of Washington and other area colleges as well as girls as young as thirteen. He was captured, tried, and convicted in Florida in 1978. Before he was killed via the death penalty in 1989, he admitted to raping, torturing, and murdering at least thirty girls and women across five states.

Laurie Olin, a graduate from the University of Washington in architecture and landscape design in the fall of 1969, lived for two months in a studio apartment at South Main and First Avenue in the heart of Skid Road. Having received funding from an anonymous donor and backing from Victor Steinbrueck and the Pioneer Square Association, he sketched and studied the people of Skid Road. He returned to the area in 1972 to continue this work before publishing his first book, *Breath on the Mirror: Seattle's Skid Road Community*.[20] Olin was raised in Fairbanks when Alaska remained a US territory. He also knew people who had moved to Alaska during the original Alaska-Yukon gold rush years.[21] Olin was familiar with the negative effects of alcohol on individuals, families, and communities, especially Indigenous communities. Although he was a highly educated young white man, it appears that Olin connected well with a diversity of people, including those who inhabited Skid Road.

Olin was surprised by the large number of disabled war veterans among the men on Skid Road, including a growing number of Vietnam War veterans, especially young Black men. The only time he encountered difficulty or the threat of violence toward him was when he tried using his camera while out on the streets. After that experience, he sketched people instead of taking photographs of them. He reported that many of the Skid Road men asked him to sketch them. One day, a young Native American man sat down next to him on a park bench and asked, "How are you at drawing scars?" Olin explained that his sketches did not always turn out well. The man replied, "There's always an impression; that's what I want to see. I want to see my impression."[22] Olin reflected on the fact that many of the Skid Road men who were either Black or Indigenous wanted him to sketch them. "These people whose identity has been brutally denied wanted to see that they were still there. My drawings seemed to reaffirm their existence."

■ ■ ■

Homelessness in Seattle and nationally underwent significant changes beginning in the 1970s and accelerating in the 1980s. Although the sprawling Hoovervilles of the Great Depression had temporarily faded into memory, the railroad hobos and tramps of previous eras still existed. What was new were the increasing numbers of homeless women, families, young adults, and runaway teens living on the streets and in emergency shelters in Seattle and other US cities. As urban planner Jill Hamberg and medical anthropologist Kim Hopper stated in a 1984 report on homelessness in America, "The suspicion is unavoidable that boundary conditions have changed, that the operating set of limits and tolerances that determines a social order's capacity to absorb surplus populations has been materially altered. Somewhere a threshold was crossed."[23]

An increase in domestic and intimate partner violence, an increase in the divorce rate, a lack of jobs, and income disparity all contributed to a deepening feminization of poverty. By the late 1970s, half of all female-headed households lived below the poverty line. It was worse for African American women and their children. There was a growing number of jobless Black men and unemployed Vietnam veterans. Many of the veterans had PTSD and heroin addictions acquired during the war. Inexpensive, highly addictive drugs, such as crack cocaine, starting in the 1980s decimated inner-city communities already living in poverty. Low-income and federally subsidized housing contracted. Welfare reform, especially under the administration of Ronald Reagan in the 1980s, cut millions of poor people from any form of public relief.

An additional factor in the rise of what became known as the "new homelessness" across the United States in the 1980s was the movement to deinstitutionalize the mentally ill. Beginning in the mid-1950s and continuing through the late 1970s, state-run, inpatient psychiatric hospitals began discharging patients back into the community. These state-run mental asylums had been progressive for their time and were protections against the abusive private contract system for the care of mentally ill people. But by the 1950s, most state mental hospitals had become overcrowded. Often, the hospital staff were abusive in their use of the newer medical and surgical procedures of frontal lobotomies, electroconvulsive therapies, and powerful antipsychotic medications like Thorazine.[24]

These problems were brought to the general public's attention by works such as Ken Kesey's 1962 novel, *One Flew over the Cuckoo's Nest*.[25] Set in an Oregon state psychiatric hospital but based on his real-life experience working in a California state psychiatric hospital, Kesey highlighted the abusiveness of the hospital system and staff like Nurse Ratched. During the shooting of the movie version (released in 1975), which was filmed at the Oregon State Hospital in Salem, Mary Ellen Mark lived in the women's ward and photographed the women inmates there as the film's still photographer. Her images of the psychiatric women inmates were published in 1979 as *Ward 81*.[26] They include intimate photographs of women taking baths and a photo of a young woman showing her scarred forearms, the crisscrossed white scars a reminder of her cutting and multiple suicide attempts.

Dorothea Dix's push in the 1850s for a direct federal role in the provision of better care for the mentally ill was finally realized in 1946 with the passage of the National Mental Health Act. This act provided grants to states to expand outpatient mental health clinics and established the National Institute of Mental Health with psychiatrist Robert Felix as its first director.[27] Felix had recently completed his master's thesis at the Johns Hopkins School of Public Health. In his thesis, he proposed a plan to replace state mental asylums with a federally funded nationwide system of community mental health centers. President Kennedy, who had a sister, Rosemary, with mental retardation worsened by a frontal lobotomy as an attempted treatment, was a proponent of a national plan to address mental retardation and mental illness. One of the last pieces of legislation Kennedy signed into law before his assassination was the Community Mental Health Act of 1963.[28]

Starting in 1966 with the opening of the first federally funded community mental health center, through 1979, 789 such centers were built across the nation. Community mental health centers were required to provide inpatient and outpatient psychiatric care, twenty-four-hour psychiatric emergency evaluations, community education, and promotion of mental health. The federal mental health program, however, never attempted to coordinate care with the state-run mental hospitals, and its service "catchment" areas did not align with local realities. Also, the civil rights movement of the 1960s and a series of significant court cases altered the involuntary confinement of psychiatric patients from a need-for-treatment standard to a standard of having to prove that the person was a danger to themselves or others.[29] The federal Community Mental Health Act, although well intentioned, was not well implemented. When Nixon was elected in 1968, he attempted to undermine the program because he equated psychiatry with communism. President Jimmy Carter, one month before his defeat by Ronald Reagan in 1980, signed the Mental Health Systems Act, hoping to save and revive the federal community mental health program. But the newly elected Reagan and the Republican-controlled Congress quickly killed the program, turning the responsibility back to the individual states to care for the mentally ill.[30]

During this time, Washington State focused more on emptying its state psychiatric hospitals than on providing robust community mental health centers. The Olmsted-designed Northern State Hospital, which in the early 1950s held 2,700 psychiatric patients, closed in 1973. More than 1,500 of its former patients had been buried in unmarked graves in a swampy area of the hospital grounds.[31] Some of its living patients were transferred to Western State Hospital, but most were discharged back into the community. A considerable number of the former patients of Northern State Hospital were given one-way bus tickets to downtown Seattle, where most of them soon became homeless.

Ironically, between 1958 and 1981, the most popular children's TV show in the Seattle area was *J. P. Patches* on KIRO. Patches, a white male tramp and clown living in a wooden shack in the Seattle city dump, was the mayor of the dump, harking back to the Hooverville days in Seattle.[32] The show included some adult humor to entertain parents and others who watched the show. Patches slept on a wood plank in his shack and ate food scraps foraged from the dump, but he had many homeless friends and appeared content with his lot in life. Erin Blackwell and other street-involved youth from the Seattle area in the 1980s likely grew up watching this show.

The popularity of J. P. Patches, the homeless, city-dump-squatting clown probably based on Charlie Chaplin's Little Tramp character of the Great Depression, likely affected people's views of homelessness in Seattle. Chaplin's direct critique of capitalism in his 1936 movie *Modern Times* led to him being put under government surveillance and then expelled from the country in 1952 during the McCarthy era. Unlike the Little Tramp, J. P. Patches did not have a subversive political message, and the show glossed over the harsh realities of poverty and homelessness in Seattle.[33]

■ ■ ■

In Seattle in the late 1970s and early 1980s, the "new homelessness" became increasingly visible. Mentally ill people who had been released from state mental institutions without sufficient housing and supportive services too often ended up on the streets, sleeping in doorways and foraging in dumpsters. So many of them ended up in the King County jail on misdemeanor charges for their survival strategies that the jail had to set up a separate psychiatric unit. A psychiatrist working there was upset by this and reportedly told a local newspaper editor, "They don't belong in a jail. They belong in a facility that can take care of them."[34] Homeless families and Vietnam veterans began to fill the available emergency shelter beds. And an increasing number of runaway teens, including Erin Blackwell, flocked to the center of the city.

Charles Royer, who was the mayor of Seattle for an unprecedented three four-year terms between 1978 and 1989, stated, "This [Seattle] is the frontier, and it's always been attractive to people. And if you go further west, you're going to get wet. Even wetter. So, it's a stopping place."[35] While mayor, Royer started the city's first task force on homelessness, which found that Seattle's existing patchwork of support services, including emergency shelters, was being overwhelmed by the increasing need.

Royer worked through the US Conference of Mayors in partnership with the Robert Wood Johnson Foundation and the Pew Charitable Trusts to address the health issues of the growing homeless populations in urban areas. In December 1983, Health Care for the Homeless, a national five-year demonstration program, was announced with an initial $25 million funding for nineteen initial demonstration projects.[36] Seattle was chosen as one of the initial projects, which was administered through the Seattle–King County Department of Health. The Health Care for the Homeless program was established mainly to test the feasibility of effective healthcare outreach to what was deemed a "difficult" and medically recalcitrant population.[37] The design of Health Care for the Homeless included, essentially, a return to the basics of public health nursing as one of the core components of the program.[38] Resisting what had become a rigidly hierarchical healthcare system, multidisciplinary teams of healthcare providers got out of the confines of the hospital and clinic and went into emergency shelters, to feeding programs, under bridges, into encampments, and onto the streets.[39]

Royer was a strong advocate for strengthening community health centers, added alcohol treatment facilities and community policing efforts, and expanded the emergency shelter system. Under Royer's administration, the Women's Advisory Board was established, which led to an increased focus on domestic violence prevention, childcare for low-income and homeless families, and increased funding for homeless youth shelters and support services.

■ ■ ■

When Erin Blackwell was first out on the streets at age thirteen, there were only two homeless youth agencies. The St. Dismas Center, a Catholic street outreach, evening drop-in center, and feeding program, was located downtown near Pike Place Market. It was a storefront space in a crumbling, old, unheated building. Above it were boarded-up hotel rooms where homeless squatters competed with rats for space.[40] Ironically, Dismas, dubbed the "Good Thief," is the Catholic patron saint of those condemned to death. The second agency serving homeless youth in Seattle then was the nonsectarian, blandly named Shelter, an eight-bed emergency shelter and drop-in center on Beacon Hill.[41] Both agencies are still in operation in Seattle. The St. Dismas Center was renamed New Horizons Ministries. It has street outreach, a youth shelter, a jobs-training program, and Street Bean Coffee, which hires former street youth as baristas. The Shelter became YouthCare, the Seattle area's largest agency serving homeless youth.

Skid Road in Seattle expanded over the years to include not only the original area south of Yesler Way, but also north along the waterfront and First Avenue to Pike Place Market and Belltown. Angeline's wooden shack, in which she lived and died, along with the other small houses of Shacktown, had been razed in the early part of the twentieth century to make way for the city's regrading efforts, expanding streets, new hotels, and a more developed waterfront. The imposing, elevated, double-decker concrete Highway 99—connecting the US-Mexico border in California with the US-Canada border in Washington State—now ran along the waterfront in Seattle. Completed in 1959 and called the Alaskan Way Viaduct, its cave-like understructure provided shelter for a growing number of homeless people.

Pawnshops, gun stores, taverns, burlesque theaters, peep shows, porn shops masquerading as bookstores, tattoo parlors catering mainly to sailors, and cheap flophouses lined First Avenue. After a summer working as a fire lookout in the North Cascades in 1956, Jack Kerouac stayed at an old $1.75/night flophouse in Skid Road in Seattle. Already an alcoholic, a disease he would die of at age forty-seven, Kerouac got drunk off cheap wine, went to a store with "girlie books," and then attended a burlesque show on First Avenue before returning to his room. In his book *Desolation Angels*, he writes that he realized he could not find a girl for the night because he was "a Skid Row bum with wine on his teeth and jeans and dirty old clothes."[42] For Kerouac, the Seattle of his imagination with its mud flats, "little shacks with seagulls," "Skid row, bars [and] Indians" became, in reality, the "sad faces of the human bars," a city where people "hang down in the unlimited void."

A former hotel for merchant sailors, which had stood near Angeline's shack along Western Avenue just below Pike Place Market, had turned into a brothel. But by the early 1980s it had been converted into low-cost housing by the Pike Place Market Foundation, housing designated for the many aging and disabled homeless and marginally housed people in the area. The foundation soon added a child daycare center, a senior day center, a food bank, a social service center, and a community health clinic.

■ ■ ■

In the late summer of 1982, when Erin Blackwell should have been preparing to begin sixth grade, she roller-skated from her mother's apartment to Pike Place Market. She already knew of the lively street scene and the hundreds of street-involved teens and young adults who hung out around the market. Many of them were what was termed "children *on* the street," meaning they had a place to live and sleep but spent most of their time on the streets. Others, including the many runaway teens, were "children *of* the street." Their entire lives were spent on or near the street, and they slept in abandoned buildings, such as old, boarded-up hotels near the market. These terms were developed by researchers and policy-makers grappling with the international phenomenon of street children, but such children and teenagers, like Blackwell, have much more complex, nuanced, and fluid lives.

A large percentage of the young people on the streets of Seattle at this time had been in the foster care system and had either run away from placements or aged out of the system. On their eighteenth birthday, they were no longer a ward of the state and were expected to take care of themselves. Despite having experienced numerous foster care placements, fractured schooling, and unaddressed significant childhood traumas, they were on their own. Many of them became homeless, and more than a few attempted or were successful in killing themselves.

From the mid-1970s through the early 1980s, the Donut House on the southeast corner of First Avenue and Pike Street across from the main entrance to the Pike Place Market was the main hangout place for homeless and near-homeless teens and young adults.[43] Its street sign proclaimed "52 Delicious Varieties" of doughnuts, and it served these doughnuts along with inexpensive coffee, hot chocolate, and soft drinks. What would become the highly lucrative Starbucks coffee company opened its first store nearby in 1971. The Donut House stayed open throughout the evening, its bright lights and large windows throwing beacons out onto the shadowy, cobblestone streets.

A young adult street outreach worker at the time, Jim Theofelis, who had grown up in the Seattle public housing project Holly Park and as a street-involved teen had become familiar with the First Avenue street scene, recalled that the Donut House was really the center of Skid Road at that time. "You'd go down there on any given night—I'm not making this up—there were 200, 300 kids." He added, "And I'd be talking to a youngster, doing outreach . . . and a car would drive up, honk the horn. The youngster would get in the car, and that was commercially exploiting teenagers. They were johns, paying johns, coming up, buying these kids."[44] The term "johns," of course, refers to the men buying sex.

Theofelis had a gun pointed at his heart one night in the alleyway behind the Donut House. The gun was held by a homeless teen he was working with, a young adolescent male, a runaway, who had been caught up in being prostituted and was using "a lot of heavy drugs" in order to deal with life. Theofelis offered him a shelter bed, and the young man drew the gun and told him to back off. "And that's when I really learned a lesson that survivors of trauma, especially youngsters, have the capacity to only manage so much goodness or attachment." Theofelis now understands that the young man was essentially saying, "I'm more comfortable getting in that car with a stranger than I am with you making me feel feelings that I don't know what to do with. . . . The last time I felt that way and trusted someone, I got hurt again. I [would] just as soon control who I get hurt by."[45]

The Donut House was a youth hangout and coffeehouse sort of model, but not exactly like the coffeehouses that Rev. Mark Matthews had in mind in the 1920s. The positive attributes were that it did not serve alcohol, and many of the street-involved youth and outreach workers remember it as a safe haven from the chaos and violence of the streets. Guenter Mannhalt owned and ran the Donut House while his brother operated a delicatessen next door.

Justin Reed Early, whose street name was "Little Justin," had run away from a foster care group home at age ten directly to the Pike Place Market. He remembered that Mannhalt was good to him. "He had a true kindness toward the kids and let us clean tables, do dishes, sweep and mop the floor in order to earn our food," Early writes in his moving memoir, *Streetchild: An Unpaved Passage*.[46] But the Seattle police did not like Mannhalt, thinking that he was up to no good and that the Donut House was a front for illegal activities. In the early 1980s, Mannhalt was charged with drug dealing and money laundering from stolen goods. Some people likened him to Fagin, the character in Dickens's *Oliver Twist*, because Mannhalt profited off his relationship with street youth in that they brought him pilfered goods from nearby stores and restaurants. Due to his continuing legal troubles, Guenter Mannhalt eventually closed the Donut House, and a Burger King replaced it.

Blackwell has reported that soon after she first roller-skated to the area, she was hooked on the other teenagers she met there, the exciting street scene around Pike Place Market, and the availability of drugs.[47] In addition, she was drawn into prostitution by forceful male pimps. Blackwell liked the money she made and the clothes, shoes, and street drugs she could buy. When she began to be prostituted, she was only thirteen and had not yet begun menstruating. She was a virgin until she made the mistake of trusting an older female street youth with that information. Her confidante informed two male pimps, who raped her while the young woman held her down. This sort of brutal "initiation" rape is all too common for vulnerable girls, young women, and young people who are LGBTQ-identified.

At age fourteen, when interviewed by Mary Ellen Mark and her husband, the documentary film director Martin Bell, Blackwell stated, "I think it is very strange that older men like little girls. They're perverts is what they is. I like the money, but I don't like them."[48] Erin Blackwell was living part of the time with her mother, who was evicted from her apartment, but increasingly was staying in cheap hotels, abandoned hotels, or squats near downtown Seattle. Blackwell also reflected on the fact that one of her "dates," which is how she referred to the men who paid her for sex, could be her father, and she would never know. Erin's mother, Pat, commenting on her knowledge that her daughter was being prostituted starting at age thirteen, calmly told Mark and Bell in an interview, "It's just a phase she's going through right now."[49]

Pimps liked underage girls working for them as prostitutes because customers often wanted young girls and because the girls rotated through the King County Juvenile Detention Center ("juvie") quickly. Adult prostitutes were arrested, kept in jail longer, and had to post bail for release. Therefore, pimps found it more lucrative to "employ" underage girls as prostitutes. In the Life magazine article on Seattle's street youth, journalist Cheryl McCall pointed out that runaway teens are especially vulnerable to survival through street prostitution. She also highlighted the fact that these youths were most often fleeing intolerable home situations, homes racked with violence, abuse, neglect, "and in a disturbingly high percentage of cases—sexual abuse."[50]

A year before the *Life* magazine story on Seattle's street youth, *Seattle Times* reporter Carol Ostrom published "Street Life Is Grim for Teen-Age Runaways."[51] Ostrom interviewed sixteen-year-old "runaway and teenage hooker" Darlene, who was prostituted at age nine on the streets of Seattle. Darlene told Ostrom that she had been raped, beaten, and stabbed while on the streets, pulling up her sweatshirt to reveal scars across her ribcage. Darlene also alluded to a history of childhood sexual abuse from which she had fled directly to the streets of Seattle. Ostrom writes, "And the pimps, stepping in where money-strapped social service agencies fail, quickly become the street kids' only support system."[52]

Changes in 1977 to Washington State's Juvenile Justice Act made it more difficult to arrest children on truancy or runaway charges. The idea was a good one: to decriminalize such juvenile offenses and strengthen the child and family welfare system. Echoing the problems that had resulted in deinstitutionalization for the mentally ill, the community support structures meant to serve as the safety net for children and families were underfunded and ineffective. Despite the change in the law, many of the street youths in downtown Seattle were arrested and placed in juvenile detention on misdemeanor charges of trespassing, jaywalking, and littering.

In her first year of being on the streets, Blackwell was arrested and kept in juvenile detention five times. Reporter Carol Ostrom interviewed a Seattle anthropologist and researcher, Deb Boyer, who estimated there were a thousand homeless youths in Seattle in 1982. "What we do," Boyer stated, "is, we take a child who's been abused—raped, neglected—we keep passing them around until they become an offender. Then we know what to do. We lock them up."[53]

Seattle officials at the time were not locking up pimps or johns—the men who were selling and buying children for sex. Pimps were arrested on drug charges but not for their key role in the sexual exploitation of girls and women. In her 1982 article, Ostrom pointed out that there had not been a single arrest of a john in Seattle the previous year. Around this time, the deputy director of the National Center for Missing and Exploited Children proclaimed that Seattle had the nation's biggest problem with juvenile prostitution, stating, "It's got to be officially sanctioned."[54]

Blackwell's frequent sexually transmitted infections—occupational illnesses of a sort—were treated at local free clinics. Washington State has the adolescent right to consent for treatment of sexually transmitted illnesses, as well as the right to access birth control at any age. The healthcare providers she saw would not have required Blackwell's mother to know about or consent for her child's medical care. Blackwell may have sought healthcare at the Seattle–King County Department of Health's VD (venereal disease) clinic downtown. But she more likely received healthcare at the Pike Place Clinic and at the Adolescent Free Clinic downtown run by University of Washington adolescent medicine physicians. Pike Place Clinic was a hippie-run free clinic.

■ ■ ■

The US healthcare system had changed by the time Blackwell was seeking treatment for her various sexually transmitted infections. America's involvement in World War II had exposed the national disgrace and negative health effects of unequal access to healthcare services. Efforts to address healthcare access at the national level finally were successful in July 1965 when President Johnson signed into law amendments to the Social Security Act. These amendments established the Medicare and Medicaid programs, both of which continue today. Medicare provides healthcare coverage to the elderly, defined as people over age sixty-five, and Medicaid provides health insurance to welfare recipients at the state level. In 1972, Medicare was expanded to include coverage for disabled people under the age of sixty-five, but only after they are disabled for two years. The two-year wait time was a Darwinian cost-saving move since more than half of all disabled people die within those two years.

When Medicare and Medicaid were first enacted, there were more than a thousand racially segregated hospitals in the country.[55] Even hospitals that were not explicitly segregated, such as most in Seattle, were de facto segregated. Besides turning away patients of color, most Seattle hospitals refused to care for people with known union affiliations through the 1950s. Harborview Hospital, King County's public hospital, was the exception because it was mandated to provide care to everyone who resided in the county regardless of race, ethnicity, socioeconomic class, or political affiliation. Medicaid and Medicare effectively ended official racial segregation in healthcare although more insidious race- and class-based health inequities continue today. Certain populations have continued to fall through the cracks of the established healthcare system. Community-based free clinics have stepped in to fill some of these gaps.

Nonsectarian free clinics, often referred to as "hippie clinics" for the people who opened and operated them, began during the 1967 Summer of Love with the Haight-Ashbury Free Clinic in San Francisco and soon spread to other urban areas, including Seattle. Based on many of the same principles as the much older people's health movement, these free clinics focused on empowering patients to care for their own and their family members' health.[56] People who opened and ran the free clinics believed that safe, accessible, and respectful healthcare was a basic human right. They believed that their free clinics would be able to phase out after universal healthcare access became a reality in the United States.[57]

Although they included physicians for the provision of primary healthcare, these clinics relied much more on social workers, nurses, ancillary medical staff, and lay volunteers. They were community-based and included community members and patients—termed "consumers"—in their governing structures. These clinics built on the grassroots advocacy and self-help organizing lessons from communist and socialist groups during the Great Depression, such as the ones Hazel Wolf had been involved with. As part of the counterculture movement of the 1960s and 1970s, hippie free clinics took care of many people experiencing the adverse effects of increased drug use, "free sex" from the sexual revolution, and the mental and physical health problems stemming from the Vietnam War. In addition, they cared for many people who were homeless.[58]

Seattle's first free clinics, both of which opened in 1968, were the Open Door Clinic and the Carolyn Downs Clinic. The Carolyn Downs Clinic, a Black Panther–run people's free medical clinic, opened in the historically African American neighborhood of the Central District. The Central District, adjacent to Yesler Terrace on First Hill, was one of the few areas of the city without racial restrictive covenants. It was not until the US Congress passed the Fair Housing Act of 1968, outlawing discrimination based on race or ethnicity in the sale or rental of housing, that these racial restrictive covenants became illegal. But illegal and enforceable are different issues. Although now illegal, racial restrictive covenants remain on many homeowner deeds in Seattle.

The Open Door Clinic was started by social worker Lee Kirschner and operated out of an old house in the University District on property owned by the University of Washington. The Open Door Clinic relied on volunteer students and faculty members from the University of Washington and had close ties with psychiatrists from the university. Ted Bundy may have been a volunteer at the Open Door Clinic since he volunteered at crisis hotlines in Seattle. The clinic, especially in its early years, did not keep good records of volunteers or patients, and whatever records existed appear to have been destroyed.

A fair number of volunteers at the Open Door Clinic were

Vietnam War conscientious objectors doing their mandatory community service. The clinic had drop-in hours and a telephone hotline staffed by volunteers and supervised by psychologists. And it had what was called the Flying Squad. The Flying Squad utilized a 1950s station wagon to transport volunteers to places around the University District and even downtown to respond to emergency calls from people on the hotline. Mavis Bonnar, one of the young volunteers on the Flying Squad, recalls that this was before the establishment in 1976 of Harborview's Medic One system, which consists of paramedic-trained firefighters being first responders to emergency calls throughout King County. Bonnar states, "The police monitored our radio waves and often arrested people before we got there. It was a different world."[59] The Flying Squad also took people to Western State Hospital in Steilacoom for direct voluntary admission.

The Open Door Clinic, at least in its early days, saw many runaway teenagers, and the staff had a network of unofficial foster homes where young people could stay. In a 1969 clinic report, which opened with Langston Hughes's poem "Genius Child," Lee Kirschner wrote that the clinic staff members were easing "the passage of this alienated group into the mainstream of our culture."[60] She concluded by writing, "As we reach more and more into a socialized and hopefully still a personalized view of physical and mental health services, Open Door will be considered an important experiment in this area." Many of the free clinics, including Open Door, were created and run under the assumption that their existence would be short-lived, that more universal access to comprehensive primary healthcare services would be implemented in the United States, thus rendering free clinics unnecessary.[61]

The clinic staff worked with churches in the University District, and a Baptist church opened its basement for overnight shelter for young people. The Open Door Clinic had a popular and welcoming living room drop-in space that even included a cat named Gleeplex, which was the brand name of a multivitamin. It was common practice at the time to hand out multivitamins to homeless people with the goal of alleviating or mitigating some of the effects of alcohol and drug abuse, as well as poor nutrition. Soup kitchen food lines often included bowls containing a rainbow mixture of multivitamins free for the taking. It was as if vitamins and bandages could cure all social ills.

A former US congressman from Washington State, Jim McDermott, was a recently graduated child psychiatrist in July 1966. He remembered that "the city was just absolutely on fire" that summer with civil rights protests over racial discrimination in housing, employment, policing, and public schools. McDermott volunteered at the Open Door Clinic until he was sent to Vietnam. Recalling his time at the clinic, McDermott said that they were seeing young people ages twelve to twenty-five who came in or were brought in by friends and who were high "on every drug imaginable."[62] Amphetamine use was the biggest problem, along with LSD, heroin, marijuana, and an unidentified substance known as the "peace pill."[63]

McDermott likened his clinical work there to the triage that he would later see on battlefields in Vietnam. At the clinic, he worked with many homeless and runaway teens, young people involved with the foster care system and juvenile detention. This work experience would later lead to his reform efforts on healthcare and on the foster care system at the state and federal levels. The Open Door Clinic struggled with funding and in the mid-1970s merged with another community-based free clinic to form the Forty-Fifth Street Clinic in Wallingford, just west of the University District. In the early 1990s, it opened an evening homeless youth and young adult drop-in clinic with funding from the Health Care for the Homeless program.

Social worker and longtime Seattle activist Joe Martin helped open the Pike Market Clinic in the former Motherlode Tavern on First Avenue in September 1978. He first worked at the First

Avenue Service Center, which was begun and run by formerly and currently homeless people. Cheap Tokay wine was the drug of choice for people in the area at that time, although marijuana and heroin were present. Martin had never seen so many tattoos before.[64] Unregulated tattoo parlors, as well as unscrupulous blood donation centers preying on homeless and poor people, would soon be identified as sources of the spread of blood-borne diseases, including hepatitis and HIV.

Pike Market Clinic had community outreach nurses who would visit patients wherever they lived, including if they were homeless on the streets, in doorways, and in encampments under the Alaskan Way viaduct. They also saw young people and may have provided healthcare or at least health advice to Erin Blackwell and other homeless and street-involved youth in the early 1980s. By then, Pike Market Clinic had moved to its current location at the north end of the market.

We know that Blackwell sought healthcare at the Adolescent Free Clinic downtown run by the University of Washington. One of her visits there was included in the documentary *Streetwise*. The clinic's outreach worker, Mavis Bonnar, and founding physician, Robert Deisher, both appear in the film and in the documentary's closing credits. This clinic was started in the early 1970s as a training program for medical students and physicians specializing in adolescent medicine. In addition to the Adolescent Free Clinic, they also operated the health clinic in the King County Juvenile Detention Center. Bonnar, who had volunteered with the Flying Squad at the Open Door Clinic in the University District, took a job as a peer outreach worker for the Adolescent Free Clinic.[65] Bonnar and the clinic physicians would have been familiar with Blackwell and many of Blackwell's street youth friends both inside juvie and in the free clinic.

The clinic physicians published some of the nation's first medical journal articles on the health of homeless teenagers. With titles such as "The Young Male Prostitute" and "The Adolescent

Female and Male Prostitute," the articles emphasize the histories of childhood physical and sexual abuse preceding adolescents' entry into homelessness and prostitution.[66] The authors point out the internalized negative stigma of being a prostitute— stigma that complicates the young person's mental health and self-concept and contributes to higher risk-taking behaviors, drug use, and suicide. Along with portraying these young people as victims, the authors also highlight the adolescents' role as disease vectors in the community, especially as the HIV/AIDS epidemic grew in the mid- to late 1980s. The emphasis on homeless youth as victims and vectors has dominated the research funding and professional literature to the present time, a deficit-only model affecting the programs and policies geared toward them.

■ ■ ■

Besides the occupational hazards of frequent arrests and sexually transmitted infections, including the newly emerging HIV/AIDS epidemic, prostituted teens like Erin Blackwell dealt with the physical and psychological hazards of rape, physical assault, and murder. By the time Blackwell began to be prostituted on the streets of Seattle, a serial rapist and murderer soon dubbed the Green River Killer had already raped and murdered five girls and young women. He had dumped their bodies in the Green River, a tributary of the Duwamish River near where the King County Poor Farm and Hospital had been located. All of them were runaways and young people prostituted along Highway 99, from near Sea-Tac Airport through downtown Seattle to Aurora Avenue North. This was a stretch of highway lined with cheap, rent-by-the-hour motels and adult sex shops.

One of the Green River Killer's earliest victims worked at a First Avenue peep show and strip joint. Another young victim disappeared from her work as a streetwalker on Aurora Avenue North. The Green River Killer, finally identified in 2001 as Gary Ridgway from south King County, was convicted of forty-eight murders. He admitted to carrying out at least seventy-one rapes and murders, saying that he lost count because there were so many. Until recently, Ridgway was America's most prolific serial killer, and he remains the country's biggest serial killer of children. The vast majority of his victims were teenagers. In addition, they were disproportionately girls and women of color, including Native Americans. That it took Seattle area police investigators so much longer to identify and arrest Ridgway than it took for Ted Bundy raises the question of whose lives are more important: the affluent, mainly white, young female college students killed by Bundy or the impoverished, runaway, homeless, prostituted, and more often nonwhite girls and young women killed by Ridgway.

A curious omission in the *Life* article and in both the book of Mary Ellen Mark's photographs and the documentary with her husband, Martin Bell, was any mention of the Green River Killer or similar dangers to Blackwell and the other prostituted teens. In the documentary, it was as if Erin Blackwell, in her street life as Tiny, was playing a real-life role of a teenage hooker along the lines of teenage Jodie Foster in the film *Taxi Driver*. But unlike the story line of *Taxi Driver*, Blackwell did not have a safe, supportive family to magically return to with the help of the PTSD-addled Vietnam veteran and New York City taxi driver played by Robert De Niro.

Mark and Bell were assisted in their work with street youth in Seattle by Teresa Kiilsgaard, a twenty-eight-year-old street outreach worker from the St. Dismas Center, now New Horizons Ministries. Kiilsgaard facilitated the *Streetwise* filming and interviews. In the *Life* magazine article, the reporter stated, "Kiilsgaard gives Erin advice, takes her for medical treatment."[67] In retrospect, I wonder about the ethical questions all of this poses. There is an element of exploitation since street youth like Blackwell were vulnerable, underage youth without any responsible parental figures in their lives. The street-involved young people were not paid for their work in the documentary film or for the use of their likenesses in the photographs. Bell would later state that they had obtained "releases" from all the people included in *Streetwise*, but what form these releases or permission forms took was never specified. And the releases likely did not include information as to the risks to the youth in terms of their participation. Did anyone explain to them that their names and images and the raw information about their young lives would be made public and perhaps haunt them for the remainder of their lives?

Mary Ellen Mark in one of her last books, *On the Portrait and the Moment*, wrote about her experiences with photographing Blackwell and other homeless young people.[68] She remembered that the *Life* journalist, McCall, "had a way of finding and demanding access to all kinds of places. She was a dynamo, like one of those little terriers that gets hold of your pants and won't let go. . . . You have to fearlessly assume you have the right to be there." In response to criticism of her photographs of street children like Blackwell and of mentally and physically disabled people as being exploitative, Mark wrote, "I hate the word *exploitive*. I think all photography is in some sense exploitive. . . . But when the word is used because I've photographed someone who is poor or disabled or just strange, it makes me angry. The people I photograph deserve to be seen."[69]

Mark and Bell both defended their work with Blackwell and the other *Streetwise* children by explaining that they were there as documentarians and not as social workers or social change agents.[70] Yet they admitted that they offered to take fourteen-year-old Tiny back to live with them in New York City when they finished filming *Streetwise* in the fall of 1983. They were in their mid-forties and childless and had grown fond of Blackwell. Their stipulation was that she go back to school. Blackwell refused and stayed living and prostituting on the streets of Seattle.

It is curious to consider this alongside information on another young homeless girl Mary Ellen Mark photographed. She photographed the Damm family in 1987 in Los Angeles for another *Life* magazine assignment. The family—a mother with two children (a school-age girl, Crissy, and a boy, Jesse), the children's stepfather, and a mean pit bull—was living in a broken-down car. Mark returned in 1994 and found them squatting illegally at a deserted ranch outside of Los Angeles. Mark walked into their room one morning and immediately took a photograph. The parents were asleep in bed, and Crissy, then just thirteen, was staring up at the ceiling in the clutches of her stepfather. Drug paraphernalia was lying on the bedside table along with a plastic statue of the Virgin Mary. Mark stated, "This is one of the most difficult photographs that I have ever taken because I felt Crissy had been abused. . . . I don't usually report my subjects to the authorities, but I reported my suspicions to a social worker assigned to the family."[71] Her suspicions were correct, and the stepfather went to prison.

■ ■ ■

Erin Blackwell's friend Justin Reed Early (Little Justin) was barely ten when he first landed on the streets in downtown Seattle. Early survived through prostitution. He did not want to be included in the *Streetwise* documentary, but he does appear in it briefly inside an enclosed phone booth at Pike Place Market. He also appears in one of Mark's photographs: a handsome, wavy-haired boy on the sidewalk clutching a giant boom box.

In his memoir, Early explains that he came from a middle-class Seattle family, but his father, a laid-off Boeing mechanic, had become an alcoholic and physically and emotionally abused Justin.[72] His mother was an alcoholic as well and did not protect Justin from the abuse. Early entered the Washington State foster care system but ran away from a group home directly to the streets of downtown Seattle. Roberta Joseph Hayes, a prostituted fifteen-year-old, befriended Early when he first appeared on the streets at Pike Place Market. She coached him on how to survive through prostitution. Early came to consider her an older sister, a key figure in his new street family. Early, Blackwell, and many other prostituted teens were lured into a dank photography studio near Pike Place Market. There, they were paid by a disheveled man to pose for nude photographs, which he sold in the lucrative child pornography industry.

Men in Seattle took advantage of street youths, especially teen girls but also boys like Justin Early. There was a robust underground network for pedophiles who shared information on where to find young prey. Homeless and runaway teens were easy targets. And there were no negative consequences for the men who purchased children for sex or who photographed them for child pornography. Perhaps they contracted the occasional sexually transmitted disease, but they were not arrested.

One of Justin Early's customers was a middle-aged married preacher from Ballard, a neighborhood north of downtown. Early even lived in this man's house for a while, with the open approval of not only the man's wife but also Early's caseworker and his parents. Using his status of being a married preacher, the man got away with sexually abusing Early. Yet this was not the worst of the system-level failures affecting the lives of Early and other street youths. Ostensibly taken out for driving lessons by King County Superior Court judge Gary Little, a middle-aged man, Early was sexually assaulted. Little was sexually abusing young boys brought before him in court. He killed himself right before the findings of an investigation were made public revealing the extent of his pedophilia. Justin Early avoided the St. Dismas outreach workers like Teresa Kiilsgaard because they all toed the line on the Catholic negative judgment of LGBTQ people. He had not fully come out yet as being gay, but he knew he "was different" and he worked as a male prostitute.[73]

Mary Ellen Mark's most famous photograph is of thirteen-year-old Erin Blackwell in a sleeveless black dress, black gloves, and black pillbox hat with a veil over her eyes.[74] Her arms are crossed defiantly—or protectively—her mouth downturned in the frown of middle age. On her chin is a prominent and subsequently permanent scar that had not been present in any of her school photographs. Was this scar from a roller-skating accident, a fight on the streets, or a physical assault from a john? Blackwell claimed she was dressed up as a "French hooker," and she appears in this same dress at the end of the *Streetwise* documentary, walking the Seattle streets, tottering on high heels.

Blackwell was the star of the documentary, coming across as high-spirited, beautiful, and smart. And she was young, unsophisticated, and poorly educated. In footage of a conversation between Erin Blackwell and Mavis Bonnar, the outreach worker for the University of Washington's Adolescent Free Clinic, Bonnar asks if Blackwell is sexually active. Blackwell asks what that means and then asks if she could be pregnant from a recent episode of sex with a "date" who refused to use a condom. Blackwell also tells Bonnar that she does not believe in abortion. She thinks she might be pregnant, and she wants a baby, "something that [is] mine, that I could say [is] mine, and I could love and do things for."[75]

■ ■ ■

Mary Ellen Mark first met Blackwell in the parking lot of a church near Pike Place Market. It was a unique church called the Sanctuary in its early days or often called the Monastery. Mainly, it was known as the "disco church." It was wood, three stories, with a square steeple, built in the early 1900s as a Norwegian immigrant Methodist church. In its life as the Monastery, its steeple at night was lit with a bright pink neon light when it was open.

The Monastery was owned and run by George Freeman, a gay Black man from eastern Washington who was in his mid-forties when he opened the church.[76] A mail-order minister in the Universal Church, Freeman claimed it was his church so he did not have to pay taxes or follow the rules in terms of sheltering teens.[77] The church basement was outfitted with hot tubs, which he called baptismal fonts. The dance floor was lit with a wild light show. Stacked amplifiers and turntables hung from the vaulted ceiling. An upper area—invitation-only—had curtained booths where sex in various forms occurred, reminiscent of the box houses of Seattle's earlier years. Freeman invited Justin Early and many of his street friends. Ecstasy was the drug of choice, although marijuana, cocaine, and LSD were prevalent as well. The Monastery was finally closed by the health department under a public nuisance statute because of concern over the "bathhouse" in the basement, which was linked with the spread of HIV/AIDS.

By 1990, HIV/AIDS was the leading cause of death in Seattle for people ages twenty-five to forty-four. The death rate from AIDS in Seattle was one of the highest in the nation. The LGBTQ community, especially gay men, was hit the hardest by the crisis. It also affected homelessness—both contributing to homelessness as people lost jobs and were evicted from homes, and disproportionately affecting people already living in homelessness. Bailey-Boushay House, an HIV/AIDS hospice, opened in 1992. The need for it was identified by people working at both the Pike Market Clinic and the Country Doctor Clinic on Capitol Hill. Capitol Hill had become a central area for Seattle's LGBTQ population. Patti, one of the prostituted teen girls in *Streetwise*, died of HIV/AIDS in 1993 at age twenty-seven.

■ ■ ■

Clearly, there were multiple systems failures for Erin Blackwell, Justin Early, Roberta Joseph Hayes, Patti, and the other children of *Streetwise*, as there still are for too many other children and adolescents. Education, healthcare, mental health and substance use counseling, the child protective system, the juvenile justice system, police, family supports—none of them worked for Blackwell. Or at least none of them worked well.

In Washington State, the Becca Bill of 1995 was enacted, amending several areas of legislation relating to truancy, at-risk youth, children in need of services, and family reconciliation.[78] The bill was named for a thirteen-year-old runaway girl from an adoptive home in Tacoma who was prostituted and brutally bludgeoned to death; her naked body was dumped in a river in Spokane. She had a long history of truancy and running away, and her foster parents felt that if Washington State had tighter laws their daughter would not have been killed. The Becca Bill was meant to give parents, guardians, and the juvenile courts more control over runaway and truant young people, ostensibly to save them from lives on the streets, prostitution, exploitation, and tragic deaths. But would the Becca Bill have altered the life trajectories of Erin Blackwell and the other street children? Likely not.[79]

The Becca Bill included mandatory reporting requirements for social workers, teachers, and healthcare providers to turn in a young person under age eighteen who was known or suspected to be homeless and a runaway. As Jim Theofelis puts it, "It really has driven kids underground. I often say that we have just empowered the pimp to be a better social worker than we are. Because we, the first thing the do-gooder says or the service provider is, 'We have to call the police, DSHS [Department of Social and Health Services], or your parents within eight hours.' Where the pimp is going to say, 'You look hungry. You look cold.'"[80]

■ ■ ■

Among the *Streetwise* youth, Patti, a prostituted teen, died of AIDS, and Duwayne hung himself in juvenile detention a few days short of his eighteenth birthday. Lulu, the ringleader of the

Streetwise young people, who was a mixed-race and openly lesbian teen, was stabbed to death by a man in an arcade on First Avenue. She was protecting her girlfriend, who was being sexually assaulted by the man who then killed Lulu. Roberta Joseph Hayes, the prostituted teen who befriended Justin Early, disappeared from the Seattle streets in February 1987. Her remains were found years later at the end of a dirt road near the Green River. She had been raped and murdered by Gary Ridgway.

Early struggled for decades with a heroin addiction, and he contracted HIV in the early 1990s while living in San Francisco. He went on to seek drug and HIV treatment and to serve on the board of directors of National Network for Youth, an organization focusing on homeless youth and young adults, with an aim to end sexual trafficking and the exploitation of young people. Early emphasizes that he is a survivor. Yet, as he points out, "Interestingly, in many ways I am still that street child. The battles and the scars remain, even though they have healed significantly."[81]

Blackwell has continued to have a difficult life yet she also survives. In the late 1980s, she began a serious crack addiction and became an alcoholic like her mother. "I cut myself when I was in my twenties. And yeah, it would take the pain away because you're not thinking about that no more, you're thinking you just sliced your arm, and now that hurts."[82] Mary Ellen Mark kept in contact with Blackwell and returned to Seattle many times to photograph her and her growing family. A photograph she took in 1993 shows a close-up of Blackwell's scarred forearms. Some of the scars appear to be track marks, and there are deep slashes on both wrists. Blackwell later acknowledged at least two suicide attempts.

Starting at age sixteen, Blackwell had ten children—five girls and five boys—with six different African American men. She is not sure who are the fathers of three of her older children. Her youngest five children are from her sixteen-year marriage to

William Charles, who was a stabilizing influence in her life. He tried to intervene with his stepchildren and teach them about being African American, including the lived experience of racism that Blackwell, being white, could not teach them. He supported Blackwell through methadone treatment.

Three of the children Blackwell had when she was still a teenager were taken into foster care. One of her younger sons is permanently mentally disabled and on SSI (Supplemental Security Income); Blackwell reveals that he is likely disabled due to her drug and alcohol consumption during her pregnancy. Her oldest daughter was arrested on prostitution charges. In 2016, Erin and Will's sixteen-year-old daughter almost died of a heroin overdose.[83] Another daughter, who says her mother used multiple drugs during her pregnancy in an attempt to abort her, is now a teacher, activist, and photographer; she is happily married and the mother of two children.[84]

Before she died in 2015 of a bone marrow disease likely caused by her long exposure to photographic chemicals, Mary Ellen Mark published a follow-up book, *Tiny: Streetwise Revisited*. Isabel Allende writes in her essay "Witnessing Tiny," which is included at the beginning of this book, "Maybe those photographs are the only constant in Erin's chaotic existence. Mary Ellen is the silent witness of her life."[85] This eloquent prose elides the fact that Mark was not silent, and it raises the question of how much and in what ways this unsilent witnessing by Mark and Bell has affected Blackwell and her children.

Blackwell, who was worried about what people would think of her and her life as exposed by the book and other follow-up to *Streetwise*, told a *Seattle Times* reporter in 2016, "I want people to think of me as being this thirteen-year-old little girl that raised myself on the streets and survived through a lot of stuff like the Green River Killer, and other people that were crazy, and through me shootin' dope and never died. Cleaning up my life and having my kids and doing the best I can do."[86] At an event at the Seattle Public Library in the fall of 2016, which included an installation of Mark's photography of Erin Blackwell as well as a screening of the newly released documentary *Tiny Revisited*, an audience member asked Blackwell what would have helped her as an adolescent to exit the street life. Blackwell, sitting on stage with three of her youngest children, thought for a moment and then replied, "Education."

■ ■ ■

Jim Theofelis, the young street outreach worker who had a gun pulled on him by a street youth in the alleyway near the Donut House, has dedicated his life to foster care and homeless youth system reform in Washington State and nationally. He was instrumental, along with psychiatrist and Congressman Jim Mc-Dermott at the federal level, in changing laws to extend foster care past age eighteen to assist youths with fractured childhoods to transition successfully to young adulthood. Theofelis, assisted by youth advocates he supported through his Mockingbird Society, successfully amended Washington State's Becca Bill with the 1999 HOPE (Homeless Youth Prevention/Protection and Engagement) Act to provide more options for homeless teens like Erin Blackwell who have no viable families to support them. He also developed the Mockingbird family cluster model of foster care, which has been adopted internationally.[87]

Noel Gomez, a prostituted teen on Seattle's streets during the time of the Green River Killer, exited the life and returned to school for a chemical dependency counselor's degree. She worked as a counselor for prostituted teens in the King County Juvenile Detention Center and then formed the Seattle-based nonprofit Organization for Prostitution Survivors. This agency includes survivor-led support services for women wanting to exit prostitution, and it also runs a men's accountability training program to educate men on the sexual exploitation of girls and women. As a society, we need to understand that prostitution is not an innocuous, victimless crime, but rather is a furthering of misogyny and violence against girls and women. Gomez knows firsthand that prostitution is "soul killing."[88]

If we can view homeless teens as more than victims and vectors and give them opportunities to not only survive but thrive, we will all be better off for that investment.

7

STATE OF EMERGENCY

As they say, history does not repeat itself, but it rhymes.

—Margaret Atwood, *The Testaments: The Sequel to the Handmaid's Tale*

Around 10:55 a.m. on an unseasonably warm and sunny late February day in 2001 in Seattle, the earth moved. First came a sound like the boom of not-so-distant thunder from the south, then steeply undulating waves, which, for someone standing on the ground outside, felt like being on a small ship in the middle of an ocean during a fierce hurricane. Utility poles swayed. Old brick buildings in Pioneer Square, including the 1899 Cadillac Hotel, crumbled, sending cascades of rubble onto the surrounding streets, which crushed cars and injured pedestrians. Car alarms screamed along with people, followed by myriad sirens from police, fire, and ambulance vehicles. A large, vintage standing clock on the sidewalk in front of the Elliott Bay Book Company in the gold rush era Globe Building stopped at the precise moment of the shaking. Water lines broke, sending geysers into the air. Soil liquefaction—where seemingly solid earth suddenly turns liquid—occurred in many areas along the Duwamish River delta, the man-made Harbor Island, and North Boeing Field in

Georgetown near where the King County Poor Farm and Hospital had been located.

What became known as the Nisqually earthquake for its epicenter in the Nisqually River delta in southern Puget Sound, was a magnitude 6.8 earthquake. The shaking only lasted forty-four seconds but seemed much longer. People still remember in detail precisely where they were and what they were doing when the earthquake struck, as they do about the September 11 attacks, which occurred seven months later on the East Coast.

More than 400 people in Seattle and the larger Puget Sound region were injured in the Nisqually earthquake, mainly from falling bricks and other pieces of old buildings. Only one person, a woman from south King County, died as a result of the earthquake. She was so frightened that she had a heart attack, and her husband could not get through to the emergency number because telephone lines were jammed. Many formerly housed people were made temporarily homeless by the earthquake, and formerly homeless but sheltered people in Seattle were made even more homeless by the disaster. Ironically, homeless people living rough outside in tents, in doorways, or under bridges that did not crumble fared best in the earthquake since their lives were not as disrupted. They were, in many ways, already living in an ongoing disaster. The American Red Cross set up emergency shelters but closed them after four days for lack of formerly housed people utilizing them. Washington governor Gary Locke declared a state of emergency and asked for federal assistance in the recovery efforts.[1]

The Compass Center in the heart of Pioneer Square on South Washington Street near the Seattle waterfront had started in 1920 as the Lutheran Sailors and Loggers Mission. In 2001, it was shelter to seventy-five homeless men but was severely damaged in the earthquake, which rendered it uninhabitable for the next four years. The nearby pier, where Alexander de Soto's Wayside Mission Hospital on the old side-wheeler and opium-smuggling

Idaho had been moored, was damaged and needed repair due to the earthquake.

The concrete pillars of the raised Alaskan Way Viaduct held, but the road required millions of dollars' worth of repairs. Engineering reports concluded that the viaduct would collapse in the event of a more direct, shallower earthquake along the Seattle fault line, which runs through the city south of Yesler Way. Engineers estimated that the viaduct would have collapsed in the deeper Nisqually earthquake if the tremor had lasted just twenty seconds more than it did. The collapse would have killed or injured hundreds of people in cars and trucks on and below the double-decker concrete highway. In addition, it would have killed and injured the many homeless people living in tents and cardboard structures underneath the viaduct. This latter fact was not included in official reports, likely because there were no city-sanctioned (allowed) encampments under the raised highway. That land was owned and maintained by the Washington State Department of Transportation. Almost immediately after the earthquake, planning began to replace the viaduct with a tunnel and a new waterfront park. The Seattle spirit of the aftermath of the Great Seattle Fire of 1889 was invoked again as the people of Seattle–King County sought to recover, rebuild, and learn from what had happened in order to prepare for future disasters.

As part of the post-earthquake disaster recovery efforts in Seattle, government officials from the Federal Emergency Management Agency (FEMA) worked with news agencies to let people know that they might qualify for federal aid if their home or apartment was badly damaged by the earthquake. Sixty homeless men who had stayed at the Compass shelter in Pioneer Square the night before the earthquake applied for FEMA aid to help with their housing. Dozens received checks of $1,200, the estimated average cost of two months' rent in Seattle at that time. Forty-three-year-old Ron Johnson, who walked with a cane and had multiple sclerosis, was paid an additional $1,000 for medication he had stored at the Compass Center and was unable to recover.

In a May 2001 *Seattle Times* article titled "Earthquake Windfall Goes to the Homeless," reporter Alex Fryer writes, "In effect, the disaster relief became a large, unexpected gift to a group of street people." He quotes Rick Friedoff, director of the Compass Center, as saying, "Some of the people who got that money weren't in the emotional frame of mind to handle it." M. J. Kiser, the Compass shelter programs manager, reported that they denied men further shelter "if they blew the money" on non–housing related expenses. Reportedly, half of the men used their FEMA money to move into permanent housing, "while others spent it on the vices of the street or squandered it." The article quotes a disgruntled homeless man who did not qualify for FEMA aid as saying that at least some of the money given to the homeless men went to "sex, drugs and alcohol." How he knew this, or if he was just making it up for the reporter, is not clear.[2] The *Seattle Times* fails to point out that no one asked formerly housed people what they spent their FEMA funds on. The language and discourse used in this article reinforced the age-old beliefs, codified by the English Poor Laws and adopted by what became the United States, that vice causes poverty and that relief, in this case in the form of FEMA funds, only deepens the misery and debauchery of the undeserving poor.

Harborview Medical Center was affected by the Nisqually earthquake not only because its staff members took care of multiple trauma cases, but also because it sustained structural damage. Earthquake retrofitting had not been completed on the 1930s art deco buildings of the main hospital and the former nurses' home, Harborview Hall, at the time of the earthquake. The hall from 1931 to 1961 had housed University of Washington nursing students who did their training at Harborview Hospital.

The building was across the street from the hospital and connected to it by an underground tunnel so the nursing students would not have to cross the street at night or in the rain.

Before the 2001 earthquake, Harborview Hall housed medical and public health researchers instead of nurses. The windowless basement held the macabre research-oriented animal euthanasia and crematorium room. On the first floor of Harborview Hall was the former nursing students' sitting room, where nurses could entertain male suitors and where they had mandatory weekly formal teas, complete with a fine china tea set and a lace cloth–covered table. The tea parties were to train the nursing students in higher socioeconomic "feminine arts," as if that was essential to the provision of quality nursing care—as if Florence Nightingale were around to still advocate for such middle-class standards. The sitting room had been converted into a King County Superior Court, where Harborview's mentally ill patients received their hearings before a judge, who decided on the need for involuntary mental health treatment.

If a modern-day insane pauper like Edward Moore had been found on the Seattle waterfront in Belltown with frozen feet in late December 2000, Medic One fire and paramedic workers would have whisked him up Profanity Hill to Harborview Medical Center, where he would have received medical care for his frozen toes—with something better than an ax sterilized with whiskey. He would have been watched over and cared for by highly skilled nurses who likely had never had tea parties as part of their education. Moore would have received a psychiatric evaluation and appeared in mental health court, where a judge would decide if he needed involuntary confinement to a state-run psychiatric facility like Western State Hospital. Hospital social workers would have attempted to find and contact his relatives in Massachusetts to see if he could be reunited with them. Moore likely would have received, or at least qualified for, after-hospital care in the supportive medical respite program associated with both Harborview and public health: Seattle–King County's Health Care for the Homeless program. This trajectory assumes that all parts of the safety net in Seattle were intact and coordinated, a best-case scenario that works for far too few people.

At the time of the earthquake, the medical respite program for homeless men was located at the Salvation Army's William Booth Center in Pioneer Square, a building that required repairs and earthquake retrofitting but that had survived the earthquake. The women's medical respite program was in the Belltown YWCA's Angeline Center, named for Kikisoblu, Chief Seattle's daughter, who had lived nearby in her wooden shack. The medical respite center for both men and women later was renamed the Edward Thomas House Medical Respite building in honor of an African American older and chronically homeless man who, in 2004, received care for leg wounds in medical respite, recovered, and was successfully housed.[3] This modern-day homeless Edward was a success story. The medical respite unit had moved to the high-rise, low-income-housing building called Jefferson Terrace, run by the Seattle Housing Authority and located across the street from Harborview's emergency department.

Harborview Hall was closed because preexisting structural instability had been made worse by the earthquake. The King County Superior Court for mental health hearings was relocated, as was the animal crematorium. Homeless people found ways into the building, and their presence was regularly noticed by security guards at night because flashlights appeared through windows. The underground tunnel connecting the hospital with Harborview Hall was redirected to connect instead with a new hospital wing. This began years of various efforts by Harborview Medical Center maintenance and security staff to secure the building, as well as more than a decade of debate by King County officials (since the county owned the property) before they could decide what to do with the building. A Harborview Medical Center master plan from 2000 had slated the building for demolition and replacement by a plaza-style park. But Harborview Hall qualified as a historic building, and architects, environmentalists, and many nurses who had trained there joined forces to save it from the wrecking ball. Environmentalists, while generally favoring the idea of more urban green space, pointed to mounting research evidence that retaining and restoring old buildings was much better for the environment than demolishing them and putting up new buildings.

Nearby Yesler Terrace, the Seattle Housing Authority's low-income housing development from the 1930s, with its 561 units of terraced, two-story, wood-frame garden apartments, was largely unscathed by the Nisqually earthquake. There were no landslides in that area, and the buildings only sustained minor damage. Even the 160-foot chimney stack at the old steam plant, which had originally supplied heat and hot water to all the housing units, survived the earthquake. But the almost thirty acres of prime Seattle First Hill real estate that Yesler Terrace was located on, with views of Mount Rainier and Puget Sound and proximity to downtown, was already targeted for upscale condominium development by Seattle multimillionaires like Paul Allen, one of the cofounders of Microsoft. First Hill was returning to its historical roots, with wealthy people moving back uphill to the area.

Disasters, whether man-made, natural, or some combination of the two, as in the case of Hurricane Katrina in the New Orleans area in 2005, always disproportionately affect poor people of color, including homeless populations. This disproportionality occurs both during the disaster or emergency and in post-disaster recovery and mitigation efforts. In Seattle post–Nisqually earthquake, for example, already scarce public and federally subsidized affordable housing was negatively impacted. Emergency shelters and transitional housing for homeless people, as well as social service support centers, are among the hardest hit by disasters since they often are located in old buildings lacking sufficient retrofitting upgrades, and they are on more undesirable, low-lying, and vulnerable land. With climate change, disasters are occurring with more intensity and with higher frequency. Efforts are underway at the federal level to address the inequities in disaster relief.[4]

When Washington governor Gary Locke—who as a child lived in Yesler Terrace with his family—declared a state of emergency on the day of the Nisqually earthquake in 2001, he was using a political and legal tool common for times of massive civil unrest or natural disaster. Declaring a state of emergency allows for the temporary revocation of certain government regulations and procedures in order to streamline and fast-track funding to address the emergency. A state of emergency also allows the temporary revocation of individual civil rights, including but not limited to the establishment of curfews and the removal and relocation of people from areas of the disaster.

■ ■ ■

On the morning of November 2, 2015, King County executive Dow Constantine and Seattle mayor Ed Murray issued a joint statement in which they declared a state of emergency in Seattle–King County for homelessness. Constantine signed a local proclamation of emergency and stated, "Emergency declarations are associated with natural disasters, but the persistent and growing phenomenon of homelessness—here and nationwide—is a human-made crisis just as devastating to thousands as a flood or fire. We call on the federal and state governments to take action, including shouldering more responsibility for affordable housing, mental health treatment, and addiction services." Constantine highlighted the racial and ethnic disproportionality of homelessness in King County: African American and Native American people were much more likely to become homeless. Murray signed a proclamation of civil emergency and pointed to a decline in federal housing support and state cuts to mental health and substance use disorder services as being major contributors to Seattle's homelessness crisis. He stated, "Cities cannot do this alone. Addressing homelessness must be a national priority with a federal response."[5]

This declaration of a state of emergency for homelessness in Seattle–King County followed similar declarations of homeless emergencies in other West Coast urban areas, including San Diego, California, and Portland, Oregon. While rates of homelessness, especially the most visible unsheltered homelessness, had been decreasing in most of the rest of the country, it was markedly increasing on the West Coast. Homelessness had become a West Coast problem concentrated along the I-5 corridor from San Diego, Los Angeles, and San Francisco, California, to Portland, Oregon, and up to Seattle, Washington.

The former western frontier cities now had the country's most robust local economies and among the highest income inequities. These cities were simultaneously the land of opportunity and plenty and the land of homelessness and despair. In the parlance of earlier times, these were cities of "tramps and millionaires" or, in modern terms, "homeless people and billionaires." Why this was and continues to be true is a matter of debate. Rapidly rising costs of housing combined with stagnant wages for entry-level and service industry jobs are most often invoked as reasons for the high rates of homelessness.[6] In Seattle, land use laws favoring single-family homes in neighborhoods reproduce the long-standing racial and ethnic segregation that began with the racial housing covenants. These laws contribute to rising housing costs. What is not mentioned is that the cities of the far West continue to draw people from other parts of the country, people in search of a better quality of life and better socioeconomic opportunities.

■ ■ ■

According to research conducted by economists Raj Chetty, Nathaniel Hendren, Patrick Kline, and Emmanuel Saez of Harvard and their colleagues with Opportunity Insights, Seattle ranks first in the nation for the probability that a child born in poverty will be able to move out of poverty by the age of twenty-six.[7] The Opportunity Insights group's aim is to apply social science and economic research to understand what helps break the cycle of intergenerational poverty. What they have found is that high-opportunity areas are that way for a host of very localized factors that are not dependent on national policies. The local city- and neighborhood-level protective factors include better public schools, higher rates of two-parent households, higher levels of civic engagement, and community cohesion. High-opportunity areas also tend to be more diverse in terms of race, ethnicity, age, and socioeconomic status. Many high-opportunity areas are not wealthy. The younger children are when moved with their family to a high-opportunity area and the longer the stay in that neighborhood during childhood, the bigger the impact.

Chetty and his group of researchers partnered with the Seattle and King County Housing Authorities to conduct a randomized controlled trial in which 421 families received housing vouchers between April 2018 and April 2019.[8] Funding was provided by the Bill and Melinda Gates Foundation. Most of the intervention group were female-headed families and nonwhite. More than a third of the household heads were immigrants. Many of the families were homeless at the time of the study, and most had histories of housing instability, including doubling up with friends and families or living in their vehicles. A large percentage of the women had experienced domestic violence and had trauma-filled childhoods. The researchers wanted to test the hypothesis that poor families would voluntarily move to higher-opportunity areas if they were provided support to reduce the barriers to doing so.

The treatment group received the help of a housing navigator from the Seattle nonprofit InterIm Community Development Association in Pioneer Square, which has a fifty-year track record of community-building work, especially with the substantial Asian Pacific Islander community and residents of Seattle's International District. The housing navigators helped the families with customized housing search assistance, negotiations with potential landlords, and language translation when needed. They also assisted the heads of household to create a "rental résumé" that included a personal essay describing their background and their hopes for the future for themselves and their children. This essay helped the housing navigators in their negotiations with landlords, especially for potential renters with poor credit histories. The housing navigators and research staff provided families with the evidence that a move to a high-opportunity area would have long-term benefits for their children. The control group families also received this information.

The individualized support for families, including fees for housing navigators and help with security deposits, cost, on average, $2,600 per family. Families in the experimental group were four times as likely as the control group families to move to high-opportunity areas of Seattle–King County. Families who moved to high-opportunity areas did so in a geographically dispersed way so as not to undermine the positive effects on a family and the neighborhood. Longer-term research is needed to understand the impacts of such moves on families and communities. The Seattle and King County Housing Authorities are planning to scale up the program.

It is worth considering what impacts such a housing program would have had on Erin Blackwell and her ten children if it had been available. Blackwell's younger children, who have had more housing and parenting stability than did her older children and have lived in higher-opportunity areas of Seattle–King County, will likely have better outcomes in life. In addition, if Blackwell had had access to the evidence-based community nurse support program, the Nurse-Family Partnership (NFP), during her first pregnancies when she was a teenager, chances are that she and her family would have had a better trajectory. Public Health—Seattle–King County has a robust NFP that pairs public health nurses with low-income, first-time pregnant young women who plan to parent their babies. The nurses follow and support the mothers and their babies through the child's second birthday. In some sense, the NFP nurses are similar to the "friendly visitors" of earlier times. Many of the NFP mothers and babies in Seattle–King County struggle with homelessness, substance use, mental health issues, and housing insecurity. The nurses help to connect them with support services and intervene with Child Protective Services in extreme cases when the mother cannot care for the child in a safe way. Although NFP was developed by David Olds, now at the Prevention Research Center for Family and Child Health at the University of Colorado Denver, Public Health—Seattle–King County was an early adopter of the program.[9]

A concern in Seattle–King County, as in many other large urban areas, is that poverty is becoming concentrated in suburban areas where housing is more affordable.[10] Social and health services, however, remain concentrated in the urban core, and that fact, combined with less public transportation in the suburbs, makes it difficult for formerly homeless people and precariously housed poor people to get to jobs and support services.

Ben Danielson, the medical director of the Odessa Brown Children's Clinic in the Central District, spoke of this issue: "King County is a suburban poverty county, and it allows us to not see as much of the poverty that's happening. It makes some of the old strategies that were from the [19]60s less relevant, and it makes some of the challenges much more difficult."[11] Danielson said that he had received a phone call the night before our November 2015 interview, alerting him to the announcement on homelessness. "Today, the King County executive and the mayor are saying that this metro area is a homelessness disaster area. That statement is really important. It's not just a sneaky way to get some federal funds pointed in some direction or another.

This is a really serious statement that's being made, especially when you think of how we're generationally affecting young people who are homeless now who are really risking being homeless for the rest of their lives."[12]

People who had worked long term in the "new homelessness" of the previous thirty years in the United States shared their view on the declaration of the state of emergency in Seattle–King County. Less than two years after the declaration, Nancy Sugg, the longtime medical director for Harborview Medical Center's Pioneer Square Clinic, reflected on her response to this news: "When a state of emergency was declared for homelessness, some of the other people that have been involved in homelessness over the years, we were all on the phone going, 'Really? It's a state of emergency?' And to me, . . . anytime you have homelessness in your city, something is just basically wrong with what's going on. Because that is, to me, such a basic human right. And when you have 10,000 [homeless] people that you count, . . . this has been a state of emergency for years, because we've been dealing with this for years."[13]

Most Americans, especially after high-profile disasters such as Hurricane Katrina, associate FEMA with large-scale crises. Less well known is the role FEMA plays in ongoing national disasters like homelessness. Since 1987, at the height of the focus on the "new homelessness" crisis across the United States, FEMA has provided funding support for emergency shelters and feeding programs for homeless people in urban areas and provided rental assistance to help prevent homelessness. Seattle–King County had been a recipient of FEMA funds for homelessness service support since the program began. Early recipients of FEMA homelessness funding in Seattle included the Downtown Emergency Service Center and the consumer-led, self-managed Tent City 1 run by Seattle Housing and Resource Effort (SHARE), both located in Pioneer Square at the time. SHARE soon merged with another self-managed community group, the Women's Housing

Equality and Enhancement League (WHEEL), to become SHARE-WHEEL. Now, SHARE-WHEEL is one of the nation's largest and longest-existing self-managed homeless programs.[14] It has built on the self-managed Hooverville in Seattle during the Great Depression and the self-help aid societies like the ones Hazel Wolf was involved with as local historical models.

The FEMA funding stream for homelessness relief is tied to certain economic metrics, including unemployment rates and the poverty levels of local communities. It does not factor in the cost of living, especially the cost and availability of affordable housing, nor the level of income inequities in metropolitan areas. Seattle–King County had received this FEMA money since it began in 1987, but in mid-2019 local agency recipients of this aid were informed the funding stream would cease. FEMA officials had disqualified Seattle–King County from receiving these funds since the official unemployment rate and poverty level had become so low.[15] Hardest hit by this funding cut has been SHARE-WHEEL, which now runs King County's largest shelter system with eleven indoor shelters, two outdoor rotating-location tent cities, and a downtown self-managed storage locker program for homeless people.

Social worker and longtime Seattle area homeless youth and young adult advocate Jim Theofelis was Mayor Murray's special advisor on homelessness at the time of the 2015 declaration of a state of emergency for homelessness. In an interview that fall, Theofelis stated, "The dilemma that I think many of us have in this field is I go home, and I'm privileged, and I close my door, and probably even [have] ice cream in the freezer. So how do I make that okay, and not shame and guilt trip my kids and family? But just stay cognizant that really how fortunate we are."[16]

Theofelis spoke of his frustrations with some vocal homeless advocates who were defending unsanctioned tent encampments around the city, including ones near Harborview Medical Center and Yesler Terrace, where tent encampment residents were preying on patients and Yesler Terrace residents. "So I have to be clear with advocates who, I think, want to say 'Everybody deserves a home!' I'm saying, 'Yeah, everyone deserves a home, and I'm going to fight as hard as I can for that. But I don't have much tolerance for robbing from poor folks. I don't have tolerance for robbing from anybody, but when you're robbing from people who are living in Yesler Terrace, yeah, I'm going to clean that up."[17] Theofelis worked as the mayor's special advisor on homelessness through the end of 2015. He went on to become the founding director of the nonprofit, public-private partnership A Way Home Washington, which is dedicated to ending youth and young adult homelessness not only in Seattle–King County, but across the state.[18]

Sociologist and Seattle homeless advocate Sinan Demirel commented, "We have a state of emergency now. But what I associate with a state of emergency is tents go up on the courthouse lawn, you know, if there's been a flood or a hurricane or something. And we're calling this a state of emergency, but it doesn't seem that we're really genuinely treating it like we would if it was housed people—clean, educated people who look and talk like us who are in this situation. We would be responding very differently." He went on to say, "In a state of emergency, in the midst of a crisis, we see structures emerge that are what we've been longing for—things that bring people together into genuine community, things that re-create civil society, like I think we used to have better in this country. Those can emerge in responding to something that's a crisis or an emergency like it really is an emergency."[19]

■ ■ ■

The Seattle–King County declaration of a state of emergency for homelessness in late 2015 came toward the conclusion of the Ten-Year Plan to End Homelessness, a project led by the Committee to End Homelessness (CEH) in King County. Officially launched in July 2005, the CEH Ten-Year Plan consisted of more than seventy businesses, county and city government officials, faith-based organizations, private philanthropists, and housing and homeless services providers. The director of the CEH, Bill Block, a prominent Seattle real estate lawyer, emphasized in meetings that Seattle–King County could end homelessness and pointed to other countries, such as Sweden, which he believed did not have homelessness.[20]

The Seattle–King County effort to end homelessness mirrored similar efforts at the federal level.[21] In 2001, President George W. Bush announced a plan to end chronic homelessness by 2012 as part of his compassionate conservatism agenda. "Chronic homelessness," although not well defined early on, refers to people who are the highest utilizers of emergency shelters, emergency departments, and other homeless and safety net services. Often, but not always, people who are chronically homeless are single adults with substance use disorders, including alcoholism, and mental health disorders, like depression and PTSD. They have multiple co-occurring physical health problems, such as diabetes, liver disease, or HIV/AIDS. They have life expectancies thirty or more years shorter than their nonhomeless counterparts. They remain homeless for long stretches of time. Critics could point to the designation of "chronically homeless" as evidence of the further medicalization of homelessness.[22] Yet anyone who works in healthcare safety net services, like public hospitals and Health Care for the Homeless programs, as well as first responders and emergency shelter frontline workers, knows that the problem is real.

In an echo back to scientific charity, national and Seattle area efforts to address homelessness, especially chronic homelessness, have highlighted the application of science, population-level surveillance, and evidence-based interventions. The federal government instituted annual point-in-time counts of homeless people, which it requires for localities to receive McKinney-Vento

Homeless Assistance grants for homeless services from the Department of Housing and Urban Development. Definitions of homelessness have differed over time and even at the same time between different agencies of the federal government. Currently, the HUD definition is the most restrictive, not counting as homeless the children in families who are living doubled-up or in temporary motel situations, while both the US Department of Health and Human Services and the Department of Education do include these children and families in their definition of homeless. Epidemiologists and survey science experts have developed methodologies for conducting point-in-time homeless counts, and the counts are now held during the final ten days of January, with the street count conducted during the early morning hours of the last Friday of the month.

In Seattle, efforts were already under way to apply research findings to create an innovative housing-first, harm reduction model to address the issue of the most entrenched chronically homeless people, the highest utilizers of public services. Housing-first harm reduction was gaining traction as an evidence-based model of care in which homeless people with substance use disorders are given safe, supportive housing without the requirement of abstinence.[23] With housing, even without treatment interventions, people often get better and reduce their use of alcohol and drugs. And often, with housing, people's mental health and physical health status improve. The national Health Care for the Homeless program had long been advocating that housing is healthcare, in an early version of the social determinants of health (SDH).[24] The SDH "are the conditions in which people are born, grow, live, work, and age that affect health" quite apart from the utilization of any healthcare services.[25] The SDH include living situations like homelessness, education and employment opportunities, neighborhood and physical environments, and social support networks.

Harborview Medical Center coordinated with the police and

criminal justice system, Medic One paramedics, Public Health—Seattle–King County's Health Care for the Homeless program, and the Downtown Emergency Service Center to identify the "chronic public inebriates" in the city who were costing the most and who were having the worst health outcomes. Amid considerable controversy but with the wide backing of city officials, the 1811 Eastlake housing project opened in 2005 in the South Lake Union area of downtown Seattle.[26] The project at 1811 Eastlake provides individual small efficiency rooms to seventy-five men and women identified by the city. The 1811 Eastlake program also maintains small cubicles on the ground floor for people who are supervised overnight. They can then be moved into one of the efficiency apartments when someone moves out or dies. Multiple studies have found significant cost savings from the program, as well as reduced alcohol intake by many of the participants.[27]

Despite the positive results noted by studies of the 1811 Eastlake program, nearby business owners and others in the community claimed that the city was paying people to be alcoholics, and the program only attracted more homeless people to Seattle.[28] This was part of the long-standing debate over what can be referred to as "don't feed the pigeons," meaning that if you provide more services for homeless people, flocks of more homeless people will come for these services. This is reminiscent of similar sentiments that were part of the Elizabethan Poor Laws.

A 1987 Los Angeles Times article titled "Original 'Skid Road'" focused on the "drunk check" and its contribution to the continued presence of homeless people in the Skid Road areas of Seattle, mainly Pioneer Square and First Avenue north to Pike Place Market. This was a monthly welfare check that Washington State paid to people who were certified unemployable because of alcoholism or drug dependency. The checks were up to $315 a month per person, and the money was supposed to go toward rent and food. People who received this "drunk check" were, on paper at least, registered in alcohol detoxification and treatment programs, but wait times for getting into those programs in King County were months long. Many people just attended Alcoholics Anonymous meetings instead. The Mayor's Task Force on Homelessness under Mayor Charles Royer recommended changes to the welfare policy, control of the sale of fortified wine such as the cheap Tokay popular at the time, and decentralization of homeless services "to break up the concentration of transients downtown." The task force instituted anti–aggressive panhandling legislation, which homeless advocates said added to the criminalization of poverty and homelessness. The *Los Angeles Times* quoted Robert Willmott, known as the "Lone Ranger of Street People," who ran a homeless feeding program in downtown Seattle, as saying, "They pay people to drink." In the article, there also was a quote from a homeless man who testified to the mayor's commission: "Seattle kind of opened its arms to street people. I got a P.O. box and an ID card and took advantage of everything here. I've been living off you guys for the last two months."[29]

■ ■ ■

For the work of the CEH Ten-Year Plan to End Homelessness, monthly meetings and community work groups were formed to focus on subpopulations of homeless people, such as veterans, families, single adults, immigrants and refugees, and youth and young adults. Many recommendations resulted from the hundreds of meetings, but the CEH lacked the authority to make policy or funding decisions. The CEH and the work groups made efforts to include homeless people's representatives, also referred to as consumers, but too often this came across as tokenism.[30] Make homelessness "rare, brief, and one time" became the federal and Seattle–King County homelessness policy-makers' mantra.

Charissa Fotinos, the former medical director of Public Health—Seattle–King County, spoke of her involvement with the CEH and her attempts to include health issues in the planning: "I think the other thing was to try and forward the conversations of the Health Care for the Homeless council. I was part of the interagency council [for] a Ten-Year Plan to End Homelessness. I participated for a couple of years, and it seemed to get to a point where what I had to offer wasn't prioritized in a way that made the most sense for me to keep going, so I switched out with someone else to fill that role. The health focus wasn't quite as large as what would have made sense to me."[31]

One of the people who had been involved with the Ten-Year Plan to End Homelessness was the new director of the CEH, Mark Putnam, who said in an interview a few weeks before the 2015 declaration of a state of emergency on homelessness in Seattle–King County, "We just created a new plan with the same goal, but we're calling ourselves All Home, with the belief and vision that all people deserve a home." He pointed out that the new name was more inclusive than the old name, and when asked what he meant by this, he replied that the name CEH was "exclusive, meaning the name itself made it seem as if there was a group of people—a committee—that was going to end homelessness, and in order to end homelessness, we need the entire community engaged. That's our belief. We need more than half, at least, of the voters to believe that all people deserve a home in order for us to achieve that vision."[32]

What precipitated the state of emergency for homelessness in Seattle–King County was the political fallout from the failure of the CEH Ten-Year Plan to End Homelessness. Although officials pointed to the 2,241 new units of affordable housing that had been built during the previous decade, homelessness in Seattle–King County had not been ended; instead, it had increased substantially.[33] One cause was the net loss of affordable housing units, including losses of housing units through the Seattle Housing Authority and the King County Housing Authority. Bill Block, Mark Putnam, and other leaders of the CEH also pointed to the effects of the housing loan crisis and the resulting Great

Recession beginning in 2007 as being reasons for the increase in homelessness and for the failure of the CEH efforts to end homelessness.

In the midst of the CEH Ten-Year Plan to End Homelessness, with the committee's focus on increasing low-income housing and pushing a housing-first agenda, the Seattle Housing Authority made plans to demolish Yesler Terrace or, as the agency put it, to "revitalize" the area and make it into a "model community."[34] By the fall of 2015, many of the Yesler Terrace housing units were demolished, and the former residents were displaced, with at least some of them becoming homeless. The area was cordoned off by temporary chain link fences, and old trees were marked as "heritage" trees for saving. One large black locust tree had a sign on it reading "Protect Tree 176, Tree Value $45,800." Double dump trucks, wrecking equipment, and large cranes dominated the area for years. Signs were posted along the busy streets of Yesler Way and Broadway proclaiming "Renewing Yesler's Promise: Building a New Urban Community," "Building Homes for All," and "Replacing Old Low-Income Housing with New."

Paul Allen and his Vulcan Corporation had made a deal with the city to develop a high-rise, luxury condominium building on the part of Yesler Terrace with the most panoramic views of Mount Rainier and Elliott Bay. The new development was called a mixed-income neighborhood, but the reality was the displacement of hundreds of former Yesler Terrace tenants and a net loss of affordable housing units.[35] The former Yesler Terrace steam plant was converted into a preschool and social services center and named the Epstein Opportunity Center in honor of Jesse Epstein, the first director of the Seattle Housing Authority. The work of Seattle social worker Irene Burns Miller in the development of Yesler Terrace has not been similarly honored.

■ ■ ■

Homelessness in Seattle–King County had not only increased dramatically in sheer numbers during the years of the CEH Ten-Year Plan to End Homelessness, but it had also changed qualitatively. There was an explosion in visible homelessness: people living in their vehicles and in unsanctioned tent encampments. Tents and tarps appeared along Yesler Way on grassy areas marked with signs saying No Trespassing / Property of King County, as well as in similar areas throughout Seattle. Ironically, a homeless encampment along Yesler Way near the I-5 off-ramp is where hundreds of units of Yesler Terrace housing had been located before I-5 came through there in the 1960s. Often located on steep hillsides along I-5 and Highway 99 (Aurora Avenue), the homeless encampments resembled the large favelas prevalent in urban areas of low-income countries.

A three-mile stretch under and around an elevated portion of I-5 beginning at Yesler Way and extending south was an area known as the Jungle. The Jungle included land where the world's largest brothel had been built in 1910 by the Hillside Improvement Company headed by the Seattle mayor and chief of police. A tough area with a high crime rate, this was an extension of the area that Jim Theofelis referred to as harboring people who stole from residents of Yesler Terrace and others around Harborview Medical Center. Tent encampments appeared in a wooded area below the medical center. A wheelchair marked Property of Harborview Medical Center was incorporated into one homeless encampment, along with dream catchers hanging from the front of a tent, soggy sleeping bags, and a tie-dyed sheet hung to dry on a temporary wire fence. Mounds of trash, cast-off clothing, and used needles lined the sidewalks nearby, including along Yesler Way. Homeless people sometimes rolled downhill into roadways. They were either too intoxicated or psychotic to know they were in danger of being run over by passing vehicles.

One of the first things Mayor Murray pushed for after the declaration of a state of emergency for homelessness was the establishment of a navigation center modeled after one in San Francisco. The Seattle Navigation Center is a low-barrier, harm reduction, pet-friendly, open 24/7, drop-in shelter with case management and rapid rehousing specialists. Based on the San Francisco model, the Seattle Navigation Center offers funds to pay people to move out of the county, supposedly to reunite with family members in other areas of the United States.[36] This is, in effect, a modern-day version of the warning-out, moving-on aspect of the English Poor Laws. It is what Seattle residents did when they literally shipped Edward Moore, the town's first official homeless person, back to Massachusetts, ostensibly to be cared for by his family. In Moore's case, it is not clear that his life was much better when he returned, and it is likely he spent at least some of the time in Massachusetts homeless before hanging himself.

Follow-up studies of homeless people who were given one-way bus tickets out of San Francisco have found that many of the people returned to San Francisco and continued being homeless, or they ended up homeless in the locations they were sent to. Planners failed to grasp the fact that many homeless people come from resource-impoverished families that are struggling with housing and food insecurities themselves.[37] Despite this evidence, in 2019 King County Council member Reagan Dunn proposed $1 million of funding to ship homeless people somewhere else. He claimed that Seattle had "become a dead-end street for the nation's homeless population."[38] But surveys included with the Seattle–King County annual point-in-time counts reveal that the vast majority of those homeless people first became homeless while living in King County.[39] Lauren McGowan, the senior director for ending homelessness and poverty at United Way King County, advocated caution in scaling up such a program as Dunn had proposed: "Just shipping someone out of town to experience homelessness somewhere else is furthering the trauma that person experiences, and furthering the crisis that we have all over the country."[40] As of December 2019, King County had included an additional $100,000 for its homeless transportation program.

Along with the Seattle Navigation Center, the mayor created the Navigation Team, which was headed by specially trained Seattle police officers who were accompanied by case managers and outreach nurses funded by Health Care for the Homeless, part of Public Health—Seattle–King County. The Navigation Team was tasked with visiting and establishing relationships with homeless people living outside in unsanctioned encampments, and then attempting to move people to the navigation center and from there into shelters or permanent housing. Often, the Navigation Team resorted to doing sweeps of the encampments—clearing them out—under public health and fire safety laws, but they encountered legal and ethical issues in doing these sweeps.[41] Critics saw the Navigation Team and its encampment sweeps as another example of the criminalization of poverty and homelessness. Also, they viewed it as an extension of the "broken windows" theory of urban disorder and decline. Based on the work of James Q. Wilson and George Kelling, broken windows theory views incivilities like panhandling, graffiti, and public inebriation "as the first harbingers of more serious crime and represent the first step on the road to urban decline."[42]

The location that Mayor Murray picked to become the navigation center, the Pearl Warren Building, already housed seventy-five homeless men through Operation Nightwatch. Rev. Rick Reynolds, the longtime director of Operation Nightwatch, stated, "We've gotten a ninety-day notice that we have to move out of there, taking our seventy-five guys out to a future we don't know. . . . Anytime there's a change to people that have fragile emotional and mental states, any minor move can be a real hazard."[43]

On the evening of January 26, 2016, Mayor Murray was giving a TV news address with an update on the state of emergency for homelessness and the proposed navigation center. At the same time, not far from the Pearl Warren Building, shootings occurred in the Jungle. Three teenage Samoan brothers, ages thirteen, sixteen, and seventeen, who were involved in the Washington State foster care system but were homeless, living together in a tent south of Pioneer Square, were charged in the murders of two people and the shooting of three more people.[44] This was allegedly a planned robbery of a Vietnamese American homeless man, well known as a drug dealer, who lived in the deepest part of the Jungle known as the Caves. The racial and immigrant/refugee issues underlying this story were palpable and roiled the tight-knit Samoan and Vietnamese communities.

The murders made the national news with headlines like "Seattle Underbelly Exposed as Homeless Camp Violence Flares" and "Slaying in 'the Jungle': Deadly Shooting at Seattle Homeless Camp Deepens Crisis." The *Washington Post* article highlighted a Seattle woman who complained about "illegally parked RVs, open drug deals and piles of needles in her Ballard neighborhood." She is quoted as saying, "The blatant lawlessness has been a whole new era." Even before the murders, social workers and outreach public health nurses had refused to go into the Jungle at any time of the day due to safety concerns. The *New York Times* article reported that Medic One paramedic firefighters would not go there without an armed police guard. It was a no man's land, a remnant of the Wild West.[45]

■ ■ ■

Frederick Jackson Turner's frontier thesis, introduced at the end of the nineteenth century at the Chicago world's fair and popularized during the early twentieth century, was based on an American amalgam of rugged individualism forged with community building, egalitarianism, and democracy.[46] One of Turner's students was Edmond S. Meany from Seattle. Meany, who dominated Seattle and Pacific Northwest history until he died of a heart attack in 1935 at the University of Washington where he taught, had more of a "booster-gatherer" approach to history. As the contemporary Pacific Northwest historian John M. Findlay describes, Meany was more concerned with "assembling and protecting the raw materials of state history" while enthusiastically and uncritically extolling the virtues of the heroic white pioneers.[47] Meany collected and preserved artifacts and oral histories of early pioneers. He even married the daughter of a pioneer he had interviewed.

Turner's American frontier thesis mainly applied to the rural, agricultural Midwest where he was from and not to the far West, which was characterized by urban, commercial, and resource extraction industrial areas like San Francisco and Seattle. Findlay contends that Washington's industrial and commercial frontiers were less individualistic, more subject to control by large corporations, more fraught with class tensions, and more prone to outbursts of violence than were the frontier regions of the Midwest. Yet Washington's, and especially Seattle's, psychological frontier was more progressive, more tolerant of, in Findlay's words, "utopians, socialists, and radicals," and more of "a malleable or open society."[48]

In Seattle, the "westering" notion of upward mobility—being able to start over and make something of oneself—to escape the decay of eastern cities was strong, at least up until the Great Depression. The extended presence of large Hoovervilles like the one near Pioneer Square in the 1930s dampened, but did not extinguish, those notions. These mythologies of place translated into the people of Seattle priding themselves on being progressive, on living in an urban area of vast opportunities, and on being egalitarian, enlightened on social issues, and capable of innovative problem solving.[49] Homelessness, especially the vast and very visible homelessness, including the new versions of

Hoovervilles, and seemingly "blatant lawlessness" that had developed in Seattle by 2015 threatened that rose-colored, progressive urban identity.

The cost of living in Seattle, especially the cost of housing, even at the higher minimum wage of $15 an hour thanks in large part to Seattle's socialist councilwoman, Kshama Sawant, first elected in 2013, means that frontline social services staff working with homeless people are often at risk of becoming homeless themselves.[50] The chaos of life on the streets and in emergency shelters retraumatizes homeless people and the frontline staff, who then suffer high rates of burnout, causing staff turnover. Talking about this problem, Rev. Rick Reynolds of Operation Nightwatch stated, "We lost a really good worker that just needed to distance themselves from it. Part of it is it's difficult work emotionally, but it also doesn't pay very well. And in Seattle's economic climate, it's tough to keep body and soul together when you're seriously underpaid."[51]

In addition to the Creating Moves to Opportunity housing voucher program, the 1811 Eastlake program, and the medical respite program, Seattle has developed other innovative programs to try to address homelessness. People working on health and homelessness issues, such as social worker Ken Kraybill, have helped develop and disseminate motivational interviewing as a more effective way to work with people, especially those dealing with substance use disorders. Motivational interviewing was first developed in the 1980s by clinical psychologists William Miller and Stephen Rollnick in their work with patients with alcoholism.[52] It was further developed by people like Kraybill for work with homeless people on a much wider spectrum of issues. Motivational interviewing focuses on building a trusting relationship with people, applying the practice of reflective listening, and supporting hope and self-direction, or, as Kraybill and Boston Health Care for the Homeless nurse Sharon Morrison put it, "helping people talk themselves into changing."[53]

Trauma-informed care was developed by people working with Health Care for the Homeless and by people working with veterans with PTSD. Ken Kraybill describes trauma-informed care as "approaches that take into account the devastating effects of particularly childhood trauma, and the impact that has on brain development and personality development and on behavior."[54]

Public health nurse Heather Barr, who began working with homeless people in the 1980s through the TB clinic in the Seattle health department before it merged with King County's health department, has worked for the Health Care for the Homeless network in Seattle–King County for more than twenty years. She visits and consults with the staff of emergency shelters and the staff and residents of tent encampments on communicable disease control and the creation of supportive environments through a trauma-informed lens. She speaks of the situation in emergency shelters as often designed to be deliberately uncomfortable. "How do we replicate or reflexively make environments look kind of like prison? Why is that? Or a harsh mental institution from yesteryear? Why is there so much cement, and how do we soften up environments so they don't seem so punitive?"[55] Barr speaks not only of trauma-informed care for individuals, but also about the roles of institutional racism and historical trauma for entire populations, especially African Americans and Native Americans. She states, "Those sorts of things probably frustrate me more and make me more upset because it's more embedded in our history and in the institutions and [in] the systems that maintain that oppression. And I guess I get frustrated sometimes when people can't grasp that concept."[56]

An additional Seattle–King County innovation that is tied to homelessness, the feminization of poverty, and gender-based violence is the regional response to the exploitation of girls and women and the Buyer Beware program.[57] Based on what is termed the Nordic model, Buyer Beware aims to increase arrests and punishments of men buying sex while decriminalizing the prostitution of women and instead connecting them with social services so they can hopefully exit the life. The buyers of sex in Seattle–King County are mainly affluent white men, while the prostituted are overwhelmingly women and girls of color and from trauma-filled and impoverished backgrounds. Sexual exploitation is a form of gender-based violence as well as a health equity issue.

The facts that Seattle is a major port city, is near the Canada-US border, and continues to support industries that mainly hire single young men all contribute to the problem of prostitution and sexual exploitation. The industries used to be logging and fishing and now are tech giants like Microsoft and Amazon. As highlighted throughout this book, the prostitution of girls and women has been normalized and made part of the authentic, gritty, Wild West cityscape of Seattle. Seattle boosters have even linked the city's history of prostitution with the Seattle spirit. In the December 1932 edition of the *American Mercury*, edited by the well-known and influential journalist H. L. Mencken, an essay titled "The Natural History of Seattle" was published. The essayist, James Stevens of *Paul Bunyan* fame, claimed that the first invocation of the Seattle spirit was when the University of Washington's first president, Asa Mercer, "imported" young white women from the Boston area. Stevens wrote about the prostitutes at the Illahee brothel in the early days of Seattle: "Every future baron or king was a worthless rapscallion until the Ill-a-hee girl fell in love with him, and made a good man out of him."[58]

Even as Seattle–King County has made progress in addressing prostitution, some people, mainly but not exclusively men, have found ways to undermine this progress. One example is the arrests of wealthy businessmen in Bellevue near Microsoft headquarters in January 2016. A group, which included high-level Amazon and Microsoft executives, such as the Microsoft director of worldwide health, was exposed as having run a private club of prostitution in a high-rise, luxury Bellevue condominium. The group called itself the League of Extraordinary Gentlemen. An Amazon software engineer who was part of the group developed an online platform for rating the "quality" of the women. He claimed that he believed this helped ensure the safety and health of the women. Most of the young women were from South Korea, did not speak English, and were lured to the United States by the men under the false pretense of being offered legitimate jobs. Then, they were kept as prostitutes and forced to sell their bodies to earn their freedom. Many of the women were raped and beaten, and a Thai woman was stabbed to death by a male customer.[59] The Seattle area has some robust groups in favor of legalizing prostitution, which are often backed by the big business that is prostitution and aided by convenient community-wide blinders as to the harm done to girls and women and the inequities that prostitution reinforces.

When she began her work as director of the Urban Indian Health Institute in Seattle in 2016, Abigail Echo-Hawk found a file folder in the bottom drawer of her desk titled "Sexual Violence." It contained results from a 2010 study conducted with researchers from the Centers for Disease Control and Prevention. The study focused on gender-based violence among Native American and Alaska Native women living in Seattle. The researchers had decided not to publish the results out of fear the study would further stigmatize an already stigmatized group of women. Echo-Hawk, along with other Native leaders in Seattle, decided to publish the results. The #MeToo movement was gaining momentum nationally, and they hoped the change would encourage people to be more supportive of the women and their stories.[60]

In the 2018 report titled "Our Bodies, Our Stories," the results of the 2010 survey of 148 Native American and Alaska Native women in Seattle found that more than half of them were homeless at the time of the survey. Nearly all the women, 94 percent, said they had been raped or coerced into sex at least once in their lives, with many of them first being raped as children or teenagers. The majority, 86 percent, said they had been negatively affected by historical trauma, including having parents or other relatives taken from their families and raised in boarding schools or sent away to distant TB sanatoriums, never to return home.[61]

Connecting with a First Nations of Canada effort, Echo-Hawk and other Native American researchers in Seattle began work on the Missing and Murdered Indigenous Women and Girls (MMIWG) advocacy project.[62] They found that in 2016 in the United States there were 5,712 missing and murdered Indigenous women, yet there were only 76 cases in the Department of Justice database. Their group surveyed seventy-one US cities that had urban Indigenous health centers and substantial numbers of urban Native American and Alaska Native residents. The city with the largest number of MMIWG cases was Seattle, with 45 documented cases. They asked cities to report on cases as far back as 1900, but the earliest documented case they found was from 1946. Even if Seattle's records had gone back to the earliest days, the death of Betsy, Kikisoblu's daughter and Chief Seattle's granddaughter, would not have been included since Betsy killed herself. Suicides of Indigenous women and girls due to domestic violence are harder to document, and they are not included in the MMIWG database.

Seattle social worker Krystal Koop is from the Makah Tribe, whose land is on the Olympic Peninsula of Washington State. She now works for the Seattle-based Partnerships for Native Health. In speaking of her own childhood in Alaska, she said, "I was homeless as a teen from the ages of twelve to fourteen in Alaska. I left my house for a lot of just alcoholism, abuse, other dysfunction, and took off and couch-surfed and slept in alleyways."[63] She was picked up by police and taken to Covenant House, the only youth shelter in Anchorage, and assigned multiple social workers through Child Protective Services. Of the

CPS social workers, she stated, "They forgot. I ended up staying at that shelter for a year, and calling CPS on my own, going, 'Where am I supposed to be? Is anybody working?'" She went on to recount how she decided then that "this doesn't work. And I would really like to be a person that I needed at that time, to follow through and communicate and let people know, give people clarity and help them navigate what is going on."[64]

Noel Gomez, who was a homeless and prostituted teen on the streets of Seattle during the time Gary Ridgway was raping and murdering girls and young women, cofounded and now directs the Organization for Prostitution Survivors in Seattle. She is working with family members of the women who were killed to have a permanent Seattle memorial for the victims of the Green River Killer. "What people don't understand is that in certain circles, it's still a huge freakin' wound," Gomez told a reporter.[65] More than half of Ridgway's victims were girls under age eighteen, and most of them were homeless. In addition, Gomez and other advocates are attempting to increase the capacity of their survivor support services. Because of the lack of capacity of these support services, combined with a massive increase in street-level prostitution along Aurora Avenue North, in the summer of 2019 police again began to arrest the women selling sex. In mid-November 2019, a fifty-three-year-old Seattle Police Department captain was arrested for sexual exploitation because he had solicited an undercover female cop posing as a young prostitute near Aurora Avenue North.[66]

Seattle city councilwoman Teresa Mosqueda, a labor Democrat first elected in 2017, focuses on health and housing inequities. She was a panelist in a public forum at the University Heights community center in the summer of 2019 focusing on city-approved vehicle residency programs, which are planned programs to support people living in their vehicles on certain faith-based or community sites. At the forum, Mosqueda spoke of the increasing number of "environmental refugees" and "water refugees" coming to Seattle to escape environmental threats like fires, droughts, and fiercer and more frequent hurricanes. Although she did not make this connection in her remarks, they conjured up memories of the environmental refugees of the Dust Bowl era, the *Grapes of Wrath* families traveling in ragged vehicles in search of jobs. The older and more derogatory term "rubber tramps" had been invoked again.

What has come to be termed "vehicle residency"—homeless and displaced people living in their cars, RVs, or even in rental moving vans—has become much more common in the Seattle area. According to the 2019 Seattle–King County point-in-time "Count Us In" report, 2,147 people were living in their vehicles on the January night of the count. To avoid parking tickets, towing, and irate housed neighbors, many people living in their vehicles try to move them around and park in public and industrial areas. In 2018, Sara Lippek, formerly a Forty-Fifth Street homeless youth clinic peer outreach worker and now an attorney, along with other lawyers with the Seattle-based Columbia Legal Services, successfully invoked the Homestead Act of 1862, when Washington was still a territory, in defense of fifty-eight-year-old Steven Long, who had been living in his truck south of Pioneer Square. "King County Superior Judge Catherine Shaffer ruled that the city's impoundment of Long's truck violated the state's Homestead Act—a frontier era law that protects properties from forced sale—because he was using it as a home," stated one newspaper.[67]

■ ■ ■

Hazel Wolf had made connections between her advocacy work with homeless and poor people during the Great Depression in Seattle and her later work with environmental issues. She credited the work of Native American environmental groups of the 1960s and 1970s with educating her on environmental justice.

She called out the health inequities for poor people of color living along the Duwamish River.[68]

Beginning in the 1970s, the lower Duwamish River was closed to fishing and swimming due to high levels of polychlorinated biphenyl (PCB) and other chemical contaminants from the industries Seattle boosters had encouraged to locate in the area. In 2001, the Environmental Protection Agency declared the area a Superfund site. In January 2019, the Navigation Team did a sweep of an unsanctioned tent encampment on a city-owned gravel lot on land where the King County Poor Farm had been located along the Duwamish River, before the river was straightened by engineers. After the sweep, environmental health inspectors found high levels of PCBs in the mud where the encampment had been located. A Seattle police officer who had been part of the Navigation Team during this sweep has sued the city for $10 million in damages, with his lawyers claiming that his exposure to PCBs contributed to health issues.[69] Exposure to PCBs has well-documented health effects, including liver damage and immune system disorders.[70]

Not widely recognized is the fact that homeless people, especially those living rough outside, are bellwethers for environmental and infectious disease threats and outbreaks that go on to affect the entire population of a community. There are, of course, instances when the actions of homeless people contribute to local environmental degradation and infectious disease outbreaks, but homeless people are more often disproportionately and earlier affected by such factors, which are beyond their control.

As Sinan Demirel framed it in 2017 in the midst of the state of emergency over homelessness in Seattle, "We have our social justice and housing activists talking one way, and our friends in the environmental movement talking another way. We just seem to be talking on parallel tracks and not lining up . . . when indeed

... the same thing that's destroying the environment is the thing that's increasing this inequality." He blamed both on a "spiritual crisis" with people "grasping for meaning in their lives, mostly out of acquiring more and more crap that they don't need and living in more and more upscale and larger places."[71]

■ ■ ■

Seattle is home to the largest United Way in the nation. Seattle–King County is home to two of the world's richest men, Bill Gates, cofounder of Microsoft, and Jeff Bezos, founder of Amazon. Seattle also is home to the nation's third-largest number of homeless people, behind New York City and Los Angeles. In terms of a per capita rate of homelessness, Seattle likely ranks first for homelessness.

A 2017 report by the *Puget Sound Business Journal* estimated that the Seattle–King County area "spends more than $1.06 billion per year addressing and responding to the homelessness crisis."[72] The researchers estimated that $119 million a year is spent in Seattle–King County on healthcare for homeless people, but that estimate only includes the cost of Medic One paramedics, uncompensated care at Harborview Medical Center, and the burial or cremation of homeless paupers. It does not include the cost of healthcare for homeless patients at other area hospitals, including Providence Hospital, nor does it include Health Care for the Homeless outreach and community health center services.

The city has allowed the construction of tiny house villages on vacant city-owned lots and contracted with the Low Income Housing Institute in Seattle to manage the villages. Now numbering ten sites scattered across the city, these tiny house villages consist of small, one-room sheds clustered around a central tent for shared meals, as well as FEMA emergency trailers containing showers and chemical toilets.[73] Sometimes derisively referred to as shacktowns, they do resemble modern-day versions of Angeline's wooden shack in Belltown. A tiny house village run by the self-managed SHARE-WHEEL near the University of Washington campus in North Seattle was ordered by the city to close down in the fall of 2019 for a lack of adequate positive outcomes of residents' entrance into permanent housing.[74] However, that decision was reversed, and the village was allowed to remain open at least through June 2020 due to concerns over transmission of the novel coronavirus in more crowded shelters.[75]

An additional $155 million a year is spent on emergency shelters and supportive housing services for homeless people. The *Puget Sound Business Journal* report quotes Craig Kinzer of real estate firm Kinzer Partners as saying about the city-approved homeless encampments, "It would be much better to build mixed income housing" on all of the sites, generating tax revenue. Kinzer, whose firm does pro bono work for Mary's Place, a women's and family shelter organization in King County, pointed out that homeless encampments, including tiny home villages, only provide temporary solutions to homelessness and frequently create ill will in the communities where they are located.[76]

Washington State has one of the most regressive tax structures in the nation, lacking both income and capital gains taxes. This leaves local governments like Seattle to rely on regressive sales taxes and property taxes for its income. Seattle has instituted some "sin taxes," such as the 2018 sweetened beverage, or soda pop, tax to raise additional funds to support food banks and other food security measures. It is not just regressive tax structures that contribute to homelessness in Seattle–King County, but also the local land use laws, which favor single-family homes, and the failure to support and protect affordable housing.

Also contributing to the homelessness problem is the continuously inadequate funding and lack of coordination of behavioral health services, including services for mental health and substance use disorders. According to Mental Health America reports, Washington has one of the nation's highest prevalence of mental illness and substance use disorders yet one of the worst behavioral health systems.[77] Wealthy people and people with private insurance can easily access excellent behavioral health services, especially in the Seattle area. Yet other people often cannot access such services, or what they can access is not responsive to their needs.

In May 2018, Western State Hospital, the state's largest and oldest psychiatric inpatient facility, failed a federal safety and quality inspection and lost federal certification and funding.[78] One of the facility's biggest problems is a lack of adequate nursing coverage due to poor salaries and working conditions, including violence by patients. Nurse and mental health reformer Dorothea Dix and Mother Joseph of the Sisters of Charity of Providence would have been livid.

In an effort to bring in more tax revenue to help address the homelessness crisis, former software engineer, socialist, and Seattle city councilwoman Kshama Sawant helped lead an effort to enact an employee hours tax, a head tax also dubbed the "Amazon tax," since it targeted large corporations like Amazon. The Seattle City Council passed the head tax ordinance in the spring of 2018, but a month later reversed its decision after Amazon threatened to halt construction on one of its new headquarter buildings in downtown Seattle and indirectly threatened to pull out of Seattle altogether.[79]

■ ■ ■

Although Seattle residents often take pride in their idea of the city being a progressive, respectful, and compassionate place, history reminds us that this has not been the case. The anti-Chinese riots and resulting expulsion of hundreds of people in Seattle in 1886 are among the more blatant examples.[80] Inevitably, in the midst of the ongoing homelessness crisis in the twenty-first century, there has been ugly and bigoted blowback.

Small-scale acts of violence against homeless people have been reported, such as a business owner in Ballard turning his hose on homeless people as they slept in their tents.[81] A Ballard town hall meeting at a church on May 2, 2018, became a shouting match as residents expressed their anger at the city for not doing more to solve the homelessness crisis, especially the homeless encampments in their neighborhood.[82] People espousing vigilante justice began videotaping homeless people and posting the content to social media in an attempt to expose and shame the visibly poor and homeless living in their midst. Tapping into the widespread anger and frustration of Seattle residents and business owners, in March 2019 Seattle's ABC affiliate, KOMO, aired the hour-long documentary *Seattle Is Dying* by reporter and former sportscaster Eric Johnson.[83]

Seattle Is Dying opens with an aerial view of a homeless encampment near what had been the Jungle along I-5; the camera pans up the hill to the tower of Harborview Medical Center and the downtown Seattle skyline. Ominous music, sounding like cardiac monitors and life support machines, plays in the background. Johnson shows people he assumes are homeless on the streets of Seattle, people he calls "wretched souls" who are "consumed by demons." He films a man eating from a garbage can on a Seattle sidewalk. Johnson asks, "How can this be who we are? How can this be what we allow? How did the word 'compassion' get twisted into this sickening reality?"[84]

Johnson makes no attempt to blur the faces of people he thinks are homeless. He concludes the documentary by offering a solution that he claims is evidence-based: take all the homeless "drug addicts" and lock them up in McNeil Island prison, located in southern Puget Sound and home to more than 200 male inmates. The inmates are all sexually violent predators who have served their prison sentences but are deemed at high risk of reoffending if released, so they live there indefinitely. Johnson claims that Seattle does not have a homelessness problem, it has a drug problem, and that Seattle elected officials are enabling widespread drug use.[85]

Seattle Is Dying became the talk of not only the Seattle area, but also nationally and even internationally.[86] The documentary was intended to be controversial and incendiary. Tim Harris, founder of the homelessness and poverty Seattle newspaper *Real Change*, called the documentary "poverty porn."[87] Catherine Hinrichsen, director of Seattle University's Project on Family Homelessness, wrote of the documentary, "It's a call to punish, rather than help, people in need, and it seeks to divide them into the 'real homeless' (or the 'deserving poor') and all the others." She concluded, "At a time when our region needs to come together on solutions, KOMO's program is a drastic, distorted, and divisive step backwards."[88]

In contrast, Anderson Cooper produced a CBS 60 *Minutes* news story on homelessness in Seattle that aired on December 1, 2019. Titled " 'Rent Is Obscene Here': The Issues Forcing People in Seattle onto the Street," this video also opens with an aerial view of a tent encampment beside I-5. Using the ambient sound of traffic instead of heart monitors, Cooper interviews a family with a three-year-old son. They are living in this approved encampment, Tent City 3, which is on city-owned property in North Seattle near the University of Washington campus. Cooper also interviews a female Seattle postal worker who works full time and is homeless; she lives in her old RV parked on a side street. She calls rent in Seattle obscene. When asked what the solution to homelessness in Seattle might be, she replies, "Affordable housing. Build it. Quit selling out to developers."[89]

In the November 2019 local elections, many Seattle and King County Council members were up for reelection, including Kshama Sawant. *Seattle Is Dying* rhetoric was invoked in many of the races. As a *Washington Post* headline reported, "Amazon Spent $1.5 Million on Seattle City Council Races: The Socialist

It Opposed Has Won."[90] Ironically, the *Washington Post* is owned currently by Jeff Bezos. Amazon had backed candidates who are more pro-business, many of whom criticized the city's response to homelessness and invoked the rhetoric in *Seattle Is Dying*. The candidates backed by Amazon money were not elected, however. Sawant is from the council district that includes First Hill, the Central District, and Capitol Hill, where Hazel Wolf lived. She is the first socialist to be elected to the Seattle City Council in the city's history. It is not a stretch of the imagination to think that Wolf, were she still alive, would have been delighted to vote for Sawant.

■ ■ ■

On the first floor of Harborview Hall, the former nurses building that was damaged in the Nisqually earthquake, a homeless shelter was opened in December 2018.[91] This was at least partially due to the early fall 2018 move by the King County Board of Health to declare homelessness a public health disaster. The board had called for an immediate increase in emergency shelter capacity before the winter months began. Before the building was converted to a homeless shelter, rooms on the first floor held emergency equipment like stretchers and neck braces, moth-eaten white physician coats, and a partial human skeleton missing arms and legs. Dirty socks and zigzagging lines of paper towel rolls lined the hallways. The shelter is operated by the Salvation Army.

In addition to the emergency shelter in Harborview Hall, the King County Council has explored ways to upgrade the old building to open a 24/7 enhanced shelter with case managers to link homeless people to housing and behavioral health services. Harborview Medical Center has primary care clinics with integrated behavioral health services.[92] In addition, the council hopes to convert upper floors into low-income and affordable housing.[93] These plans have been put on hold due to the coronavirus pandemic public health emergency, which was declared by Seattle mayor Jenny Durkan and King County executive Dow Constantine. Harborview Hall was turned into a forty-five-bed COVID-19 recovery site for people without homes who need supportive care.[94] In effect, Harborview Hall and Harborview Medical Center have become a modern-day version of the original King County Poor Farm and Hospital in Georgetown.

Harborview Medical Center, which started out so long ago as the King County Poor Farm and Hospital first run by the Sisters of Charity of Providence, has become not only a medical refuge for homeless and impoverished people of King County, but also a beacon of hope for critically injured and ill people across a four-state region. Seattle has long been called the best city to have a heart attack in and survive. Harborview Medical Center physicians, such as Michael Copass, and the Medic One system in Seattle–King County he helped develop are the reason for the good survival rates for a heart attack. Copass, who was the director of emergency services at Harborview for thirty-five years before retiring in 2008, trained generations of physicians and paramedics to treat every patient, even the smelliest and most belligerent homeless patient, with respect. "I used the force of righteousness. I called everybody who was admitted to the ER a 'gold coin.' I just didn't want to see anybody mistreated. Nobody grows up to be a bum. And so we didn't have any bums, we only had gold coins. We did not have GOMER—'grand old men of the ER,' which is a phrase coined at Harborview—or 'get out of my ER.' We just had gold coins."[95]

One of the paramedics and then emergency services physicians whom Copass trained is David Carlbom. Carlbom works at Harborview Medical Center and is the director of the Michael K. Copass MD Paramedic Training Program there. Carlbom remembers one evening in the apparatus bay in the Medic One fire station, which is part of Harborview's emergency department.

Copass said to Carlbom, "'Stop just a second. Maybe you've figured this out, but maybe you haven't.' He told me that there's a river of love that flows underneath this place. And the way to do better, and to continue to do better, and be a force for good, is to connect to that river of love. And that is the magic of this place."[96]

■ ■ ■

People in Seattle–King County agree on one thing: there is a problem, a state of emergency, with homelessness. But they don't agree on the precise reasons for the rise in homelessness in Seattle–King County, much less the solutions. Homelessness is a wicked problem. "Wicked" public problems are unstructured, crosscutting, and relentless. They are complex and multifaceted, "engendering a high degree of conflict because there is little consensus on the problem or the solution."[97] A wicked problem like homelessness "is not going to be solved once and for all despite all the best intentions and resources directed at the problem."[98] Wicked problems also confound science-based understanding. They are the "swampy lowlands" of urban planner Donald Schon's striking statement about the high, hard ground of professional practice, where "manageable problems lend themselves to solution through the use of research based theory and technique."[99] But, he warns, this high, hard ground overlooks a swamp where "problems are messy and confusing and incapable of technical solution." He points out the irony of this situation: the problems of the high ground are relatively unimportant, "while in the swamp lie the problems of greatest human concern."[100]

Both homelessness and the US healthcare system are considered prime examples of wicked problems. So is climate change. When considering healthcare issues for homeless people in the United States and in Seattle–King County, it seems to become a swamp from a policy, planning, and political perspective, and it is also a swamp filled with quicksand, or perhaps it's a Superfund swamp.

The King County CEH Ten-Year Plan to End Homelessness, which became All Home, continues to have no authority over policies and no funding mechanism, although efforts are under way to change that. In January 2018, Mayor Durkan, along with King County executive Constantine and the mayor of Auburn in south King County, Nancy Backus, formed One Table.[101] One Table, a name reminiscent of King Arthur's Knights of the Round Table, included business leaders, homeless service providers, and university researchers, who were tasked with identifying the root causes of homelessness in the Seattle–King County region.

In a series of three meetings over six months, One Table identified five root causes of homelessness: a lack of affordable housing, inadequate access to behavioral health services, negative impacts on youth in the child welfare system, negative impacts for people with prior involvement with the criminal justice system, and education and employment gaps.[102] But One Table dissolved almost as quickly as it had been formed.

■ ■ ■

Murray Morgan ends the updated edition of his *Skid Road*: "The only certainty is that Seattle will continue to change. The salt water that laps the pilings of the waterfront opens onto the oceans of the world. The mountains still catch and hold the rain of the eastering winds. The scenery is better than if it had been planned. Dead peaks come to life. New dreams continue to form."[103] In a prescient and still-current encapsulation of Seattle's history, he writes, "The mood is transitory. Seattle has known other moments of hesitation, of pauses that depressed. They have been followed, quite often, by outbursts of energy in unexpected directions, . . . by the sudden unity of a community of disparate people."[104]

Although Morgan makes it sound as if Seattle has bipolar disorder, he draws on his deep knowledge of the city's history to emphasize people's ability to find common ground on issues that otherwise divide. Despite the ongoing state of emergency for homelessness in Seattle–King County, as long as we continue to invoke the spirits of practical mystics, the intrepid men and women we mistook as being voiceless, as long as we tap into the river of love and muck about in the swamp together, we can address health and social inequities in radical and innovative ways.

HEARING VOICES

As I went walking, I saw a sign there,
And on the sign there, it said "no trespassing."
But on the other side, it didn't say nothing,
That side was made for you and me.
—Woody Guthrie, "This Land Is Your Land"

In the early fall of 2017, a homeless man moved into my backyard. I will call him Mike. I knew Mike from seeing him around the Seattle campus of the University of Washington where I work, but I did not know him personally. He slept in doorways of buildings on campus, including near the Health Sciences Library, and he wandered around during the daytime, carrying a ragged backpack and talking to himself. He seemed harmless and lonely and sad.

First, Mike dragged an old mattress from a nearby house and placed it in my backyard. A neighbor told me that the mattress had been thrown out because it had bedbugs. I had not realized that Mike thought my house was his until the day I discovered he had taped a large, official No Trespassing: Private Property sign to my front door. He likely took the sign from a nearby business.

That same day, he threatened to shoot the man who was repainting the outside of my house. He pointed toward the sign on my front door and told the man he was trespassing. A neighbor, a woman who works at the city jail, heard Mike's threat and called the police. Mike had wandered across the street to the fire station by the time the police arrived. Mike accused the police officer of trespassing and asked the firefighters to arrest the officer.

Mike was arrested and sent to Harborview Medical Center for inpatient psychiatric treatment. What became of him after that, I do not know, but I have not seen him around campus or near my house. My neighbor who works at the city jail told me that Mike has a long history of homelessness, arrests for criminal trespassing, and psychiatric treatment at both Harborview and Western State Hospital—but he is regularly discharged back into the churn of chronic homelessness in Seattle. He has a family in Washington State, including siblings and two grown children, but he has burned his bridges with all of them and is now on his own.

Seattle's plan to bus homeless people out of town to their families would not work for Mike. Perhaps by now he has benefited from obtaining supportive permanent housing, including community-based mental health treatment, and that is why I no longer see him on the streets or around campus. I prefer to think that is true versus the alternative options, including that he was among the hundreds of homeless people who died outside in 2019 in Seattle–King County.

One of those people who died outside in 2019 was another homeless man in the University District and Capitol Hill area in Seattle. William Kaphaem, who preferred to be called Three Stars in honor of his Mohawk ancestry, was found dead and "skeletonized" in the bottom of the fourteen-foot aluminum rowboat he called home.[1] The rowboat was anchored near the end of the failed Empire Expressway and the "bridges to nowhere" from the late 1950s in the Washington Park Arboretum on Lake Washington. Three Stars was fifty-nine years old. Curled up beside him and also dead in the boat was his little dog, Buddy. They were found in late August 2019 after a complaint to the authorities by a man walking through the park.

The King County medical examiner determined that Three Stars had died of natural causes—most likely hypothermia—during the cold winter months of 2018–2019. Three Stars was from Massachusetts but had lived in Seattle since 1980 and had worked as a street performer downtown, playing his guitar and singing country songs. He had been homeless for at least a decade and was on Social Security disability for a mental illness that he said he had had since childhood. In 2011, he told a *Seattle Times* reporter that he lived in a rowboat because he liked living close to nature and said, "I've got a lot of stuff. I don't want to schlep it around town like some tramp."[2] Three Stars was estranged from his family.

I think of mental health reformer Dorothea Dix's plea for "seasonable care," the early identification and treatment of mental illness. We now know that for most mental illnesses, especially schizophrenia, depression, and bipolar disorder—as well as for childhood trauma and substance use disorders—seasonable care does have the best long-term outcomes for the individual and for society. Three Stars lived homeless—and died homeless—largely because of untreated mental illness. And Mike grew up in and is now chronically homeless with a mental illness in a state with one of the worst mental health systems in the United States. Mike has received inpatient treatment on numerous occasions from Western State Hospital, a mental facility that has been decertified and defunded by the federal government due to its poor quality of care. Efforts are under way to resurrect and strengthen community-based mental health in the state and in Seattle–King County, harking back to the national, state, and local efforts in the 1960s—efforts that failed and contributed to the rise in "new homelessness" beginning in the 1980s. I hope we do better this time.

Although I experienced homelessness myself as a young adult due to underlying childhood traumas, mental health challenges, job loss, divorce, and breaks with my family of origin, I now benefit from the privilege of being an educated white woman with a decent job and health insurance that includes mental health coverage. I can afford to be a "worried well" patient whenever I choose to be one. I now own a house in Seattle that I can afford to have repainted. This is at least partially due to the intergenerational transfer of wealth since my parents were white and owned their home. I can afford to live, and I have raised my children in a relatively high-opportunity area with access to good public schools, great public libraries, and reasonably high levels of social cohesion and of diversity.

The episode of Mike moving into my backyard literally brought home to me the multiple issues of homelessness in Seattle–King County, issues that I was researching and writing about as I prepared this book. It is much easier to keep the wicked problem of homelessness at an emotional arm's length when a homeless person has not moved into your patch of backyard, your personal space. Or when you have not experienced homelessness yourself. I was, of course, reminded of Hazel Wolf and her involvement during the Great Depression in the Federal Theatre Project play in Seattle *One-Third of a Nation*, based on Franklin Roosevelt's speech about one-third of the nation living in substandard housing. I was reminded specifically of the play's opening scene with the character of a founding father standing on a patch of grass and holding a sign proclaiming, "This is mine / Keep off." Who am I—who are any of us—to own land in Seattle, the ancestral land of the Duwamish tribe?

I admire the work of Seattle architect Rex Hohlbein, his daughter Jenn LaFreniere, and other people at the Seattle nonprofit

Facing Homelessness who help match homeless people, including mothers with small children, with homeowners who have built backyard dwellings for them. Called the Block Project, it has the motto "Yes, in my backyard," as opposed to the usual "not in my backyard" approach. It requires the buy-in of people in the neighborhood, or at least the city block, where a formerly homeless person will live.[3] The organization's aim is to have a homeless person or family supported by an entire community, recognizing that homelessness is not just "houselessness" as many advocates now claim. Homelessness is about the lack of interpersonal affiliations, connections, and supports that make a house a home. Although this is not something I can see myself doing anytime soon, I like that the Block Project and Facing Homelessness exist in my city. It gives me hope that we can become better versions of ourselves and create a better version of our city.

In this, I am reminded of the words of Rev. Craig Rennebohm, who began a still-thriving street-based mental health outreach program for homeless people in Seattle.[4] "I realized that if we can't bring some level of peace to our neighbors on the streets, in our communities, there's no hope for us being a more peaceable presence in the world. We need to learn how to be peaceable and healing at the most fundamental levels of our common life—as families, as neighbors, as cities and towns—communities."[5]

■ ■ ■

The same month that Mike moved into my backyard, I began a new position as director of the Doorway Project at the University of Washington, a multimillion-dollar state-funded project tasked with "ending youth homelessness in the University District." I was working on the design of a community café model instead of a navigation or homeless drop-in center as a more effective way to address youth and young adult homelessness, including among University of Washington students.[6] The Doorway Project is part of the university's Homelessness Research

Initiative, bringing together researchers from different disciplinary silos to try to solve the problem of homelessness.

I did not want to use the Doorway Project funding for the usual endless planning meetings or needs assessments, something we are prone to do in academia. I also did not want to use the funding for anything like the Ten-Year Plan to End Homelessness of which I had been a part through my role as a primary care provider for homeless youth. I did not want the Doorway Project to be just another extractive research project to "study the problem of youth homelessness." I was not interested in writing and publishing another academic journal article. And I had the luxury of both tenure and seniority to be able to opt out of that usual requirement of the "high, hard ground" of academic research.

I wanted to muck about creatively in the swamp of the wicked problem of homelessness. I wanted action and what I thought of then as innovation—the development and opening of a social enterprise in the form of a community café that was welcoming to everyone but that unobtrusively could help to connect young people to needed health and social supports. I sought to create a community café that could help address the stigma of homelessness, that would allow for a third space, a safe space for community members to have unsafe conversations about hard topics like racism, classism, trauma (including historical trauma), gender-based violence, mental illness, and substance use disorders. This community café would counter the narrative that claimed "Seattle is dying." But the coffeehouse model was not so innovative or new after all, as I discovered through my research for this book.

In the two years I worked as the director of the Doorway Project, our team planned and conducted seven pop-up community café events in the University District, events that included participatory planning with young people to help create the more permanent café. But I also encountered significant political and institutional challenges I had not anticipated and for which I ran out of patience. We were not able to open a community café. So, at the end of two years, I handed over the leadership of the Doorway Project to someone more adept at dealing with the inevitable compromises associated with such endeavors. I now believe that a nimbler, mission-driven, grassroots, community-based nonprofit like Facing Homelessness would have a better chance of opening and sustaining the community café that I envisioned.

■ ■ ■

What I learned through the research and writing of this book helped me become more patient in some ways and less patient in others. I'm less patient with people who use homelessness as a political tool for their personal gain. Less patient with myself when I find that I fall into that category. Less patient with the seemingly never-ending and toothless versions of the Ten-Year Plan to End Homelessness, All Home, One Table, and whatever comes next. Less patient with the homelessness industrial complex that Seattle–King County and the United States supports in the interest of charity over justice and solidarity in any form. Less patient with myself for being part of that homelessness industrial complex and continuing to benefit from it. Less patient with the perpetuation of violence against women and children and people of color. Less patient with our collective intolerance of opposing viewpoints and of people we see as "other" in all its permutations.

At the same time, through this project I became more patient with people and with entire communities who struggle to survive and thrive despite seemingly insurmountable obstacles. I became more patient with myself for continuing to learn the lessons of endurance—and resistance.

Although I am not a historian, through this book project I learned that history teaches us to take the long view. Positive change takes time. It also takes collective effort. As one of my mentors, Seattle retired social worker Nancy Amidei, reminded me as she reflected back on the changes she has lived through, including the start of Medicare and Medicaid, food stamps, Head Start, the Civil Rights Act, the Americans with Disabilities Act, and Title IX: "If you have lived through that kind of change and you've seen it happen—and most of that is stuff that helps people who are not rich, are not powerful—food stamp recipients are not rich and powerful, welfare moms are not rich and powerful—we can do things in this country, and you don't have to be rich and powerful to make it happen. But you do have to vote, and you do have to pay attention to who's in office. You do have to pay attention to the candidates, and you do have to speak up—and care. You don't have to be an expert, you just have to care."[7]

Through this project, I learned, in the words of historian David Hitchcock, that history training is "empathy training (among other things)."[8] Many of the people whose lives I have pieced together and presented in this book captivated me. Even though most of them are long dead, they drew out the "feeling with," the mirrored emotion that is a central facet of empathy, versus the colder, more at arm's-length sympathy. I wrestled with the thorny ethical issues of digging up the dirt and delightful relics, and I have told the stories of mostly forgotten, overlooked, and largely voiceless people, like Edward Moore and Kikisoblu. I feel strongly that these are, in Seattle poet Claudia Castro Luna's words, "mute voices / that need to be heard."[9]

Coll Thrush, writing about the Indigenous history of Seattle, reminds us that stories matter, especially the palimpsest of place-stories that can lead to a better understanding of history and, in turn, to constructive, collective action. "These place-stories . . . will not simply be cautionary tales, smug jokes, or nostalgic fantasies, but will be dialogues about transformations of landscape and power in the city and about strategies for living together in this place." He encourages us to listen to new stories to inform "new kinds of action."[10]

Wicked problems like homelessness will not be solved by any of the science or policy schemes of the high, hard ground upon which we too often stake our claim. Wicked problems like homelessness are best approached by being willing to enter the swamp, to value the role of stories, of a multiplicity of stories, and to nurture the capacity to listen to—and for—them. We must especially listen to the quieter voices telling their stories, or even mere fragments of stories.

ACKNOWLEDGMENTS

Many people and institutions supported my research and writing of this book. I would like to thank historian Lorraine McConaghy for her mentorship, friendship, and guidance throughout this project. My son, Jonathan Bowdler, who is completing his doctorate in history, also provided important perspectives and resources that were essential for the completion of this book. My thanks extend to the many people who graciously gave their time for oral history interviews and shared their experiences and views of homelessness and healthcare in Seattle–King County. My Skid Road Oral History interviews (video- and audiotaped) and transcripts will be stored at the University of Washington Libraries, Special Collections, for future researchers to access.

The dedicated and patient librarians at various institutions were essential to my work. I thank librarians at the Seattle locations of the Museum of History and Industry, Providence Archives, King County Archives, Seattle Public Library, and the University of Washington Libraries, Special Collections. At Providence Archives in Seattle, Emily Dominick (now the head of Special Collections Technical Services at the University of Washington Libraries, Special Collections) and Elizabeth Russell, associate archivists, and Peter Schmid, visual resources archivist, were helpful to me. In addition, Sister Rita Bergamini, founder of the Providence Archives, was gracious in sharing with me her stories of having worked as a nurse at Providence Hospital beginning in the 1940s.

Lisa Oberg, associate director of History of Science and medicine curator at the University of Washington Libraries, Special Collections, was a key resource. Anne Davis, anthropology librarian at the University of Washington Odegaard Library, assisted me with a photography and video exhibit and panel discussion about my Skid Road project from December 2017 through February 2018. Lynly Beard, research impact and social work librarian at the University of Washington Health Sciences Library, has been an ongoing source of information and support for my work. For my research on the English and Scottish Poor Laws, I want to thank the librarians at the British Library in London and the National Library of Scotland in Edinburgh for their assistance. The reference librarians at Worcester Public Library in Worcester, Massachusetts, assisted me in tracking down the official death register of Edward Moore.

I am grateful for the sanctuary of public libraries and for the understanding and compassionate librarians in my local library who are kind to a homeless woman pushing her cart of possessions through the lobby and washing her face in the bathroom. Seattle has numerous little free libraries around houses and schools. In one of these close to my home, I found and read an exquisitely beautiful handmade journal written by an older homeless woman. Although I decided for ethical reasons that I could not use her journal as source material for this book, I want to thank this anonymous woman for sharing her insights about the lived experience of homelessness in Seattle–King County. I have returned her journal to the little free library so others may read it and hopefully pass it on.

Thank you to Claudia Castro Luna, Seattle's first civic poet (2015-2017) and Washington State's poet laureate (2018-2020), for granting permission to use part of her powerful "Seattle's Poem" as the epigraph for this book. "Seattle's Poem" is included in her anthology *This City* from Floating Bridge Press.

My work on this book was made possible through a US-UK Fulbright Award, the University of Washington's Walter Chapin Simpson Center for the Humanities, the National Endowment for the Humanities, Humanities Washington, 4Culture Heritage Projects, and the Jack Straw Cultural Center.

Thank you to the anonymous reviewers of early drafts of the manuscript, as well as to Robin Coleman, acquisitions editor at Johns Hopkins University Press, for helping guide the final version of this book. I want to extend a special thanks to my copyeditor, Merryl A. Sloane, who provided me with expert advice on the final draft of the manuscript.

I am grateful to my nursing colleagues Drs. Maggie Baker, Marla Salmon, Teresa Ward, Amy Walker, and Elaine Walsh for their continued support of my writing and public scholarship. Thank you to the members of my writing group, the Shipping Group, and to our group's founder and leader and my writing mentor, Waverly Fitzgerald, for support and guidance. Waverly died after a brief illness in December 2019, but her nurturing spirit lives on in the wide writing community she was part of. I extend special thanks to my writing partner, Mary Oak, for her helpful critiques of early drafts of chapters of this book. In addition, I want to thank Karen Maeda Allman, longtime bookseller and author events coordinator at Elliott Bay Book Company in Seattle, for her support of my work.

My family, including my son, Jonathan; my daughter-in-law, Lily; my stepdaughter, Margaret; and my new granddaughter, Hazel, provided support, grounding, and delight. This book is dedicated to my partner, Peter Kahn, for his unwavering enthusiasm and support of my research and writing.

NOTES

PROLOGUE. ONE WOMAN'S SEATTLE

1. Murray Morgan, *Skid Road: An Informal Portrait of Seattle*, 2nd ed. (1982; repr., Seattle: University of Washington Press, 2018).

2. King County, "Medical Examiner's Office–Investigated Deaths among People Living Homeless," March 3, 2020, https://www .kingcounty.gov/depts/health/examiner/services/reports-data/ homeless.aspx.

3. Coll Thrush, "Hauntings as Histories: Indigenous Ghosts and the Urban Past in Seattle," in *Phantom Past, Indigenous Presence: Native Ghosts in North American Culture and History*, ed. Colleen E. Boyd and Coll Thrush (Lincoln: University of Nebraska Press, 2011), 54–81, 54.

4. Coll Thrush, *Native Seattle: Histories from the Crossing-Over Place*, 2nd ed. (Seattle: University of Washington Press, 2017).

5. Morgan, *Skid Road*, 9.

6. Morgan, 9.

7. David Lavender, *Land of Giants: The Drive to the Pacific Northwest, 1750–1950* (Lincoln: University of Nebraska Press, 1979).

8. Nicholas St. Fleur, "Earliest Known Human Footprints in North America Found on Canadian Island," *New York Times*, March 28, 2018, https://www.nytimes.com/2018/03/28/science/footprints-oldest-north -america.html.

1. Coll Thrush, *Native Seattle: Histories from the Crossing-Over Place*, 2nd ed. (Seattle: University of Washington Press, 2017).

2. David M. Buerge, *Chief Seattle and the Town That Took His Name: The Change of Worlds for the Native People and Settlers on Puget Sound* (Seattle, WA: Sasquatch Books, 2017); Clarence Bagley, *History of King County, Washington* (Seattle, WA: Clarke Publishing, 1929); Frederic James Grant, ed., *History of Seattle, Washington, with Illustrations and Biographical Sketches of Some of Its Prominent Men and Pioneers* (New York: American Publishing and Engraving, 1891), http://hdl.handle.net/2027/wu.89067417691; Roberta Frye Watt, *The Story of Seattle* (Seattle: Lowman and Hanford, 1931).

3. Watt; John Caldbick, "Henry Yesler's Steam-Powered Seattle Sawmill Cuts Its First Lumber in March 1853," *HistoryLink*, August 1, 2014, http://www.historylink.org/File/760; Kathie Zetterberg with David Wilma, "Henry Yesler's Native American Daughter Julia Is Born on June 12, 1855," *HistoryLink*, July 30, 2001, https://www.historylink.org/File/3396.

4. Murray Morgan, *Skid Road: An Informal Portrait of Seattle*, 2nd ed. (1982; repr., Seattle: University of Washington Press, 2018), 36.

5. Richard Burn, *The History of the Poor Laws: With Observations* (Clifton, NJ: Kelley, 1973); David Hitchcock, *Vagrancy in English Culture and Society, 1650–1750* (London: Bloomsbury, 2016).

6. Walter I. Trattner, *From Poor Law to Welfare State: A History of Social Welfare in America*, 6th ed. (New York: Free Press, 1999).

7. William P. Quigley, "Reluctant Charity: Poor Laws in the Original Thirteen States," *University of Richmond Law Review* 31, no. 1 (1997): 111–78.

8. David Hitchcock, "'Punishment Is All the Charity That the Law Affordeth Them': Penal Transportation, Vagrancy, and the Charitable Impulse in the British Atlantic, c. 1600–1750," *New Global Studies* 12, no. 2 (2018): 195–215, 195–96, https://doi.org/10.1515/ngs-2018-0029.

9. Hitchcock.

10. Hitchcock, 200.

11. John Winthrop, *A Modell of Christian Charity* (1630), https://history.hanover.edu/texts/winthmod.html.

12. Trattner, *From Poor Law to Welfare State*.

13. Quigley, "Reluctant Charity."

14. Mary De Young, *Madness: An American History of Mental Illness and Its Treatment* (Jefferson, NC: McFarland, 2010).

15. Quigley, "Reluctant Charity."

16. Edith Abbott, "Poor Law Provision for Family Responsibility," *Social Service Review* 12, no. 4 (1938): 598–618.

17. Legislative Assembly of the Territory of Washington, An Act Relating to the Support of the Poor, Laws of Washington, 1854–1862, Washington State Library, Olympia.

18. King County Washington Commissioners, *Beginnings, Progress and Achievement in the Medical Work of King County, Washington* (Seattle, WA: Peters Publishing, 1930); Marion Hathway and John Rademaker, *Public Relief in Washington, 1853–1933: Poor Relief, Mothers' Pensions, Indigent Soldiers' Relief, Old Age Pensions, and Indigent Blind Relief in Washington* (Olympia: State of Washington Emergency Relief Administration, 1934).

19. Morgan, *Skid Road*.

20. John M. Hunter, Gary W. Shannon, and Stephanie L. Sambrook, "Rings of Madness: Service Areas of 19th Century Asylums in North America," *Social Science and Medicine* 23, no. 10 (1986): 1033–50, https://doi.org/10.1016/0277-9536(86)90262-5.

21. Dorothea Lynde Dix, *Asylum, Prison, and Poorhouse: The Writings and Reform Work of Dorothea Dix in Illinois* (Carbondale: Southern Illinois University Press, 1999).

22. Thomas J. Brown, *Dorothea Dix: New England Reformer* (Cambridge, MA: Harvard University Press, 1998).

23. Dix, *Asylum, Prison, and Poorhouse*.

24. Kathleen Jones, *The Making of Social Policy in Britain, from the Poor Law to New Labour* (London: Athlone, 2000).

25. Tamonud Modak, Siddharth Sarkar, and Rajesh Sagar, "Dorothea Dix: A Proponent of Humane Treatment of Mentally Ill," *Journal of Mental Health and Human Behaviour* 21, no. 1 (2016): 69–71, https://doi.org/10.4103/0971-8990.182088; Dorothea Dix, "'I Tell What I Have Seen': The Reports of Asylum Reformer Dorothea Dix," *American Journal of Public Health* 96, no. 4 (April 1, 2006): 622–24, https://doi.org/10.2105/AJPH.96.4.622; Dorothea Lynde Dix, *The Lady and the President: The Letters of Dorothea Dix and Millard Fillmore* (Lexington: University Press of Kentucky, 1975).

26. Brown, *Dorothea Dix*.

27. Nancy Rockafellar and James W. Haviland, eds., *Saddlebags to Scanners: The First 100 Years of Medicine in Washington State* (Seattle: Washington State Medical Association, Education and Research Foundation, 1989).

28. Brown, *Dorothea Dix*.

29. Dix, *Asylum, Prison, and Poorhouse*.

30. Brown, *Dorothea Dix*, 90.

31. Thomas Wickham Prosch, "The Insane in Washington Territory," 1914, Pacific Northwest Historical Documents Collection, PNW00694, University of Washington, http://digitalcollections.lib.washington.edu/cdm/ref/collection/pioneerlife/id/3651.

32. Judith Walzer Leavitt and Ronald L. Numbers, *Sickness and Health in America: Readings in the History of Medicine and Public Health*, 3rd ed. (Madison: University of Wisconsin Press, 1997).

33. Prosch, "Insane in Washington Territory."

34. Prosch.

35. Prosch, 4.

36. Prosch.

37. Legislative Assembly of the Territory of Washington, An Act Relating to the Support of the Poor, 1.

38. Prosch, "Insane in Washington Territory," 4.

39. Prosch, 5.

40. Prosch.

41. Trattner, *From Poor Law to Welfare State*; Quigley, "Reluctant Charity."

42. Lorraine McConaghy, *Warship under Sail: The USS Decatur in the Pacific West* (Seattle: Center for the Study of the Pacific Northwest in association with University of Washington Press, 2009).

43. Thrush, *Native Seattle*.

44. Wolfgang Jilek, *Indian Healing: Shamanic Ceremonialism in the Pacific Northwest Today* (Blaine, WA: Hancock House, 1982); Wolfgang Jilek, *Salish Indian Mental Health and Culture Change: Psychohygienic and Therapeutic Aspects of the Guardian Spirit Ceremonial* (Toronto, ON: Holt, Rinehart and Winston, 1974); Wolfgang G. Jilek and Norman Todd, "Witchdoctors Succeed where Doctors Fail: Psychotherapy among Coast Salish Indians," *Canadian Journal of Psychiatry* 19, no. 4 (1974): 351–56, https://doi.org/10.1177/070674377401900404; Roxanne Dunbar-Ortiz,

An Indigenous Peoples' History of the United States, repr. ed. (Boston: Beacon, 2015).

45. J. Neilson Barry, "Archibald Pelton, the First Follower of Lewis and Clark," *Washington Historical Quarterly* 19, no. 3 (1928): 199–201.

46. Barry; "Franchère's Narrative of a Voyage to the Northwest Coast, 1811–1814," Library of Congress, accessed June 23, 2018, https://www.loc.gov/item/04036133/.

47. Morgan, *Skid Road*.

48. Prosch, "Insane in Washington Territory," 6.

49. Ezra S. Stearns, *History of Ashburnham, Massachusetts, from the Grant of Dorchester, Canada, to the Present Time, 1734–1886, with a Genealogical Register of Ashburnham Families* (Ashburnham, MA: published by the town, 1887), http://archive.org/details/historyofashburnoostea.

50. Stearns.

51. Ancestry.com, *Massachusetts, Death Records, 1841–1915*.

52. Stearns, *History of Ashburnham, Massachusetts*, 544–45.

CHAPTER 2. SKID ROAD

1. E. Meliss, "Siwash," *Overland Monthly and Out West Magazine* 20, no. 119 (November 1892): 501–6, http://name.umdl.umich.edu/ahj1472.2-20.119.

2. Julia Anne Allain, "Duwamish History in Duwamish Voices: Weaving Our Family Stories since Colonization," PhD diss., University of Victoria, 2014, https://dspace.library.uvic.ca//handle/1828/5790.

3. Roberta Frye Watt, *Four Wagons West: The Story of Seattle* (Portland, OR: Binfords and Mort, 1931); Thomas Wickham Prosch, *David S. Maynard and Catherine T. Maynard: Biographies of Two of the Oregon Immigrants of 1850* (Seattle, WA: Lowman and Hanford Stationery and Printing, 1906).

4. Matthew W. Klingle, *Emerald City: An Environmental History of Seattle* (New Haven, CT: Yale University Press, 2007).

5. Quintard Taylor, *The Forging of a Black Community: Seattle's Central District from 1870 through the Civil Rights Era* (Seattle: University of Washington Press, 1994).

6. Nancy Isenberg, *White Trash: The 400-Year Untold History of Class in America* (New York: Viking, 2016).

7. Isenberg.

8. Frederick Jackson Turner, *The Frontier in American History* (New York: Holt, 1920), https://archive.org/details/frontierinamericooturnu-oft/page/n4/mode/2up.

9. Watt, *Four Wagons West*; Thomas Stowell Phelps, *Reminiscences of Seattle, Washington Territory, and the U.S. Sloop-of-War "Decatur" during the Indian War of 1855–1856* (Seattle, WA: Alice Harriman, 1908), http://hdl.handle.net/2027/yale.39002005686457.

10. Phelps.

11. Junius Rochester, "Conklin, Mary Ann (1821–1873) aka Mother Damnable," *HistoryLink*, January 1, 1999, https://www.historylink.org/File/1934.

12. Lorraine McConaghy, *Warship under Sail: The USS Decatur in the Pacific West* (Seattle: Center for the Study of the Pacific Northwest in association with University of Washington Press, 2009), 141.

13. David M. Buerge, *Chief Seattle and the Town That Took His Name: The Change of Worlds for the Native People and Settlers on Puget Sound* (Seattle, WA: Sasquatch Books, 2017).

14. Buerge.

15. Allain, "Duwamish History in Duwamish Voices."

16. Buerge, *Chief Seattle and the Town That Took His Name*.

17. David Blaine, *Memoirs of Puget Sound: Early Seattle, 1853–1856: The Letters of David and Catherine Blaine* (Fairfield, WA: Ye Galleon Press, 1978), 17.

18. Blaine, 135–36.

19. Blaine, 120–21.

20. Coll Thrush, *Native Seattle: Histories from the Crossing-Over Place*, 2nd ed. (Seattle: University of Washington Press, 2017).

21. McConaghy, *Warship under Sail*.

22. McConaghy.

23. Alexandra Harmon, *Indians in the Making: Ethnic Relations and Indian Identities around Puget Sound* (Berkeley: University of California Press, 1998).

24. Dennis W. Johnson, *The Laws That Shaped America: Fifteen Acts of Congress and Their Lasting Impact* (New York: Routledge, 2009).

25. Mary E. Odem, *Delinquent Daughters: Protecting and Policing Adolescent Female Sexuality in the United States, 1885–1920* (Chapel Hill: University of North Carolina Press, 1995).

26. Buerge, *Chief Seattle and the Town That Took His Name.*

27. Kathie Zetterberg with David Wilma, "Henry Yesler's Native American Daughter Julia Is Born on June 12, 1855," *HistoryLink*, July 30, 2001, https://www.historylink.org/File/3396.

28. Philip Joseph Deloria, *Indians in Unexpected Places* (Lawrence: University Press of Kansas, 2004).

29. Deloria.

30. Blaine, *Memoirs of Puget Sound.*

31. Charles Prosch, *Reminiscences of Washington Territory: Scenes, Incidents and Reflections of the Pioneer Period on Puget Sound* (Seattle, WA: n.p., 1904), 27, 124, http://hdl.handle.net/2027/njp.32101078192562.

32. Taylor, *Forging of a Black Community.*

33. Thrush, *Native Seattle.*

34. Thrush.

35. James W. Haviland, "The Broad Sweep: A Chronological Summary of the First 100 Years of Medicine and Dentistry in Washington State, 1889–1989," in *Saddlebags to Scanners: The First 100 Years of Medicine in Washington State,* ed. Nancy Rockafellar and James W. Haviland (Seattle: Washington State Medical Association, Education and Research Foundation, 1989), 1–26, 3.

36. Murray Morgan, *Skid Road: An Informal Portrait of Seattle,* 2nd ed. (1982; repr., Seattle: University of Washington Press, 2018), 5.

37. Coll Thrush, "Hauntings as Histories: Indigenous Ghosts and the Urban Past in Seattle," in *Phantom Past, Indigenous Presence: Native Ghosts in North American Culture and History,* ed. Colleen E. Boyd and Coll Thrush (Lincoln: University of Nebraska Press, 2011), 54–81, 63.

38. Thrush, *Native Seattle.*

39. Priscilla Long, "Madame Lou Graham Arrives in Seattle in February 1888," *HistoryLink*, January 1, 2000, https://www.historylink.org/file/2762.

40. A. Atwood, *Glimpses in Pioneer Life on Puget Sound* (Seattle, WA: Denny-Coryell, 1903), 89, http://hdl.handle.net/2027/wu.89072934342.

41. Thrush, *Native Seattle,* 131.

42. Thrush, 131.

43. Allain, "Duwamish History in Duwamish Voices."

44. Robert William Summers, *Indian Journal of Rev. R. W. Summers: First Episcopal Priest of Seattle (1871–73) and of McMinnville (1873–81)* (Lafayette, OR: Guadalupe Translations, 1994), 1–2.

45. Buerge, *Chief Seattle and the Town That Took His Name*.

46. "Angeline Won't Go," *Seattle Post-Intelligencer*, March 16, 1890, 8.

47. Buerge.

48. Summers, *Indian Journal of Rev. R. W. Summers*, 242.

49. Bertha Piper Venen, *Annals of Old Angeline: "Mika Yahoos Delate Klosch!"* (Seattle, WA: Denny-Coryell, 1903).

50. David Lewis, "The Man Who Burned Down Chief Seattle's Lodge," *Seattle Weekly*, August 25, 2016, https://www.seattleweekly.com/news/the-man-who-burned-down-old-man-house/.

51. "Holy Things, Holy People: The Rosary of Princess Angeline," St. James Cathedral, June 8, 2014, https://www.stjames-cathedral.org/history/holythings/10angeline.aspx.

52. "Princess Angeline Is Dead," *New York Times*, June 1, 1896.

53. Venen, *Annals of Old Angeline*.

CHAPTER 3. THE SISTERS

1. Ellis Lucia, *Seattle's Sisters of Providence: The Story of Providence Medical Center, Seattle's First Hospital* (Seattle, WA: Providence Medical Center, Office of Public Affairs, 1978).

2. Thomas Wickham Prosch, "A Chronological History of Seattle from 1850 to 1897," 1900, typewritten manuscript in Thomas Wickham Prosch Papers, University of Washington Special Collections, Seattle.

3. Thomas Wickham Prosch, *David S. Maynard and Catherine T. Maynard: Biographies of Two of the Oregon Immigrants of 1850* (Seattle, WA: Lowman and Hanford Stationery and Printing, 1906).

4. Prosch, *Chronological History of Seattle*.

5. King County Washington Commissioners, *Beginnings, Progress and Achievement in the Medical Work of King County, Washington* (Seattle, WA: Peters Publishing, 1930), 11.

6. King County Washington Commissioners, 13.

7. King County Washington Commissioners, 23.

8. Margaret Humphreys, *Malaria: Poverty, Race, and Public Health in the United States* (Baltimore, MD: Johns Hopkins University Press, 2001).

9. Coll Thrush, *Native Seattle: Histories from the Crossing-Over Place*, 2nd ed. (Seattle: University of Washington Press, 2017).

10. Thrush.

11. Prosch, *David S. Maynard and Catherine T. Maynard*; Paula Becker, "Maynard, Catherine Broshears (1816–1906)," *HistoryLink*, March 3, 2004, http://www.historylink.org/File/4281.

12. Dorothea Nordstrand, "Doc Maynard: Seattle Pioneer," *History-Link*, January 20, 2004, http://www.historylink.org/File/4273.

13. Nordstrand.

14. King County Washington Commissioners, *Beginnings, Progress and Achievement*.

15. Terri Mitchell, "The King County Poor Farm: Origin of Providence and Harborview Medical Centers," *Columbia: The Magazine of Northwest History* 16, no. 2 (June 2002): 8–14.

16. Sister Mary McCrosson of the Blessed Sacrament, *The Bell and the River* (Palo Alto, CA: Pacific Books, 1957).

17. McCrosson.

18. McCrosson.

19. Nancy Rockafellar and James W. Haviland, "The Broad Sweep: A Chronological Summary of the First 100 Years of Medicine and Dentistry in Washington State, 1889–1989," in *Saddlebags to Scanners: The First 100 Years of Medicine in Washington State*, ed. Nancy Rockafellar and James W. Haviland (Seattle: Washington State Medical Association, Education and Research Foundation, 1989), 1–26.

20. McCrosson, *The Bell and the River*.

21. McCrosson.

22. Thomas Wickham Prosch, "The Insane in Washington Territory," 1914, Pacific Northwest Historical Documents Collection, PNW00694, University of Washington, http://digitalcollections.lib.washington.edu/cdm/ref/collection/pioneerlife/id/3651.

23. Russell Hollander, "Mental Health Policy in Washington Territory, 1853–1875," *Pacific Northwest Quarterly* 71, no. 4 (1980): 152–61.

24. Hollander.

25. Walter I. Trattner, *From Poor Law to Welfare State: A History of Social Welfare in America*, 6th ed. (New York: Free Press, 1999).

26. Oscar R. Ewing, "History of the United States Public Health Service, 1798–1948," *Public Health News* 29, no. 9 (1948): 275–78.

27. Edmond Stephen Meany, *History of the State of Washington* (New York: Macmillan, 1909).

28. McCrosson, *The Bell and the River*; Ezra Meeker, *Pioneer Reminiscences of Puget Sound; The Tragedy of Leschi; An Account of the Coming*

of the First Americans and the Establishment of Their Institutions; Their Encounters with the Native Race; The First Treaties with the Indians and the War That Followed; Seven Years of the Life of Isaac I. Stevens in Washington Territory; Cruise of the Author on Puget Sound Fifty Years Ago; Nisqually House and the Hudson Bay Company (Seattle, WA: Lowman and Hanford Stationery and Printing, 1905).

29. Lucia, Seattle's Sisters of Providence; Sophie Frye Bass, When Seattle Was a Village (Seattle, WA: Lowman and Hanford, 1947).

30. "Catechism of the Catholic Church: The Virtues," accessed May 21, 2019, http://www.vatican.va/archive/ccc_css/archive/catechism/p3s1c1a7.htm.

31. David Blaine, Memoirs of Puget Sound: Early Seattle, 1853–1856: The Letters of David and Catherine Blaine (Fairfield, WA: Ye Galleon Press, 1978).

32. Gene Balk, "Washingtonians Are Less Religious Than Ever, Gallup Poll Finds," Seattle Times, April 20, 2018, https://www.seattletimes.com/seattle-news/data/washingtonians-are-less-religious-than-ever-gallup-poll-finds/.

33. Hollander, "Mental Health Policy in Washington Territory."

34. Chronicles and patient ledgers, Sisters of Providence Archives, Seattle, WA.

35. Chronicles.

36. Chronicles.

37. Chronicles.

38. Mitchell, "King County Poor Farm."

39. Chronicles and patient ledgers, Sisters of Providence Archives.

40. Michael B. Katz, In the Shadow of the Poorhouse (New York: Basic, 1986).

41. Ruth Richardson, Dickens and the Workhouse: Oliver Twist and the London Poor (New York: Oxford University Press, 2012).

42. Michel Foucault, Discipline and Punish: The Birth of the Prison (New York: Vintage, 1979), 204–5.

43. Trattner, From Poor Law to Welfare State.

44. Richardson, Dickens and the Workhouse.

45. Richardson, 3.

46. Trattner, From Poor Law to Welfare State.

47. Raphael Hulkower, "From Sacrilege to Privilege: The Tale of Body

Procurement for Anatomical Dissection in the United States," *Einstein Journal of Biology and Medicine* 27, no. 1 (March 2, 2016): 23–26, https://doi.org/10.23861/EJBM20112734; Michael Sappol, *A Traffic of Dead Bodies: Anatomy and Embodied Social Identity in Nineteenth-Century America* (Princeton, NJ: Princeton University Press, 2002).

48. Norman M. Keith and Thomas E. Keys, "The Anatomy Acts of 1831 and 1832: A Solution of a Medical Social Problem," *AMA Archives of Internal Medicine* 99, no. 5 (1957): 678–94, https://doi.org/10.1001/archinte.1957.00260050006002; Steven Robert Wilf, "Anatomy and Punishment in Late Eighteenth-Century New York," *Journal of Social History* 22, no. 3 (1989): 507–30.

49. Ruth Richardson, *Death, Dissection, and the Destitute* (London: Routledge and Kegan Paul, 1987).

50. James Gerald Crowther, *Statesmen of Science: Henry Brougham, William Robert Grove, Lyon Playfair, the Prince Consort, the Seventh Duke of Devonshire, Alexander Strange, Richard Burdon Haldane, Henry Thomas Tizard [and] Frederick Alexander Lindemann* (Chester Springs, PA: Dufour, 1966), 9.

51. Kenneth C. Nystrom, "Postmortem Examinations and the Embodiment of Inequality in 19th Century United States," *International Journal of Paleopathology* 1, nos. 3–4 (2011): 164–72, https://doi.org/10.1016/j.ijpp.2012.02.003.

52. Sappol, *Traffic of Dead Bodies.*

53. Kristina Killgrove, "How Grave Robbers and Medical Students Helped Dehumanize 19th Century Blacks and the Poor," *Forbes*, July 13, 2015, https://www.forbes.com/sites/kristinakillgrove/2015/07/13/dissected-bodies-and-grave-robbing-evidence-of-unequal-treatment-of-19th-century-blacks-and-poor/.

54. Department of County Poor, King County, Coroner's Cremation Transfer Forms, Coroner Pre-1969, 1726 216-1-2, King County Archives, Seattle, WA.

55. J. Tate Mason, "Biennial Report of the King County Hospital, 1917–1918," ser. 147, box 6, King County Archives, Seattle, WA.

56. Florence Nightingale, "On Trained Nursing for the Sick Poor," *Times* (London), April 14, 1876.

57. Nightingale.

58. Diana C. Archibald and Joel J. Brattin, *Dickens and Massachusetts:*

The Lasting Legacy of the Commonwealth Visits (Amherst: University of Massachusetts Press, 2015); Jenny Hartley, *Charles Dickens and the House of Fallen Women* (London: Methuen, 2009).

59. Hartley.

60. Providence Hospital Seattle and Pacific Northwest Catholic History Collection, *The Golden Sheaf: A Short Sketch of Providence Hospital, Seattle, Washington: Golden Jubilee Years, 1877–1927* (Seattle: n.p., 1927).

61. Anna Clare Duggar, "Providence Hospital, 1877–1909," 1948, typewritten manuscript, Providence Archives, Pacific Northwest History Collection, Seattle, WA.

62. Providence Hospital Seattle and Pacific Northwest Catholic History Collection, *Golden Sheaf*.

63. *Chronicles* and patient ledgers, Sisters of Providence Archives, Seattle, WA.

64. "The Baby Mystery Solved," *Daily Intelligencer*, November 8, 1879.

65. "Baby Mystery Solved."

66. *Chronicles* and patient ledgers, Sisters of Providence Archives.

67. "Jumped the Town," *Daily Intelligencer*, November 28, 1879, 3.

68. *Chronicles* and patient ledgers, Sisters of Providence Archives.

69. Barbra Mann Wall, *American Catholic Hospitals: A Century of Changing Markets and Missions* (New Brunswick, NJ: Rutgers University Press, 2011).

70. Barbra Mann Wall, *Unlikely Entrepreneurs: Catholic Sisters and the Hospital Marketplace, 1865–1925* (Columbus: Ohio State University Press, 2005), 163.

71. Lucia, *Seattle's Sisters of Providence*, 56.

72. Lucia, 56.

73. Junius Rochester, "Prefontaine, Father Francis Xavier (1838–1909)," *HistoryLink*, December 2, 1998, https://historylink.org/File/3633.

74. *Chronicles* and patient ledgers, Sisters of Providence Archives.

75. Mitchell, "King County Poor Farm."

76. *Chronicles* and patient ledgers, Sisters of Providence Archives.

CHAPTER 4. ARK OF REFUGE

1. Malcolm McDonald, "The Samaritan Spirit—Seattle's Pharisees," *Commonwealth*, May 23, 1903.

2. McDonald; Irving Safford, "De Soto's Descendant and His Proposed Christian Work," *Seattle Post-Intelligencer*, July 31, 1898.

3. McDonald; Safford.

4. Rebecca Anne Allahyari, *Visions of Charity: Volunteer Workers and Moral Community* (Berkeley: University of California Press, 2000).

5. Norris A. Magnuson, *Salvation in the Slums: Evangelical Social Work, 1865–1920* (Metuchen, NJ: Scarecrow, 1977).

6. K. Steven Vincent, "Elie Halevy on England and the English," *Modern Intellectual History* 12, no. 1 (April 2015): 173–96, https://doi.org/10.1017/S1479244314000407.

7. Jacob August Riis, *How the Other Half Lives: Authoritative Text, Contexts, Criticism* (1901; repr., New York: Norton, 2010).

8. Riis, *How the Other Half Lives*; Jacob A. Riis, *The Children of the Poor* (1890; repr., New York: Sagwan Press, 2015).

9. Jacob August Riis, *The Making of an American* (New York: Macmillan, 1916).

10. "The Omaha Platform: Launching the Populist Party," *History Matters*, accessed July 8, 2019, http://historymatters.gmu.edu/d/5361/.

11. David B. Williams, *Too High and Too Steep: Reshaping Seattle's Topography* (Seattle: University of Washington Press, 2015).

12. David M. Buerge, *Seattle in the 1880s* (Seattle, WA: Historical Society of Seattle and King County, 1986).

13. Buerge.

14. Marion Hathway and John Rademaker, *Public Relief in Washington, 1853–1933: Poor Relief, Mothers' Pensions, Indigent Soldiers' Relief, Old Age Pensions, and Indigent Blind Relief in Washington* (Olympia: State of Washington Emergency Relief Administration, 1934), 11–12.

15. Hathway and Rademaker, 12.

16. Charles E. Rosenberg, *The Cholera Years: The United States in 1832, 1849, and 1866*, 2nd ed. (Chicago: University of Chicago Press, 1987).

17. Quintard Taylor, *The Forging of a Black Community: Seattle's Central District from 1870 through the Civil Rights Era* (Seattle: University of Washington Press, 1994).

18. Buerge, *Seattle in the 1880s*.

19. Robert Wynne, "Reaction to the Chinese in the Pacific Northwest and British Columbia, 1850 to 1910," PhD diss., University of Washington, 1964 (ProQuest).

20. Charles Pierce LeWarne, *Utopias on Puget Sound, 1885–1915* (Seattle: University of Washington Press, 1995).

21. Carlos A. Schwantes, *Radical Heritage: Labor, Socialism, and Reform in Washington and British Columbia, 1885–1917* (Seattle: University of Washington Press, 1979).

22. John Rankin Rogers, *Free Land: The Remedy for Involuntary Poverty, Social Unrest and the Woes of Labor* (Tacoma, WA: Tacoma Morning Union, 1897).

23. Rogers.

24. Richard White, *A New History of the American West: "It's Your Misfortune and None of My Own"* (Norman: University of Oklahoma Press, 1991), 434–35.

25. Schwantes, *Radical Heritage*.

26. "Klondiker's Souls," *Evening Journal*, November 9, 1897; "Bound for the Klondike," *Evening Star*, November 24, 1897.

27. "Scenes in the Wayside Mission," *Seattle Post-Intelligencer*, September 3, 1899.

28. "Klondiker's Souls," 2.

29. Irving Safford, "De Soto's Descendant and His Proposed Christian Work," *Seattle Post-Intelligencer*, July 31, 1898.

30. "Klondike Evangelists," *Seattle Post-Intelligencer*, June 30, 1898.

31. Margaret Humphreys, *Malaria: Poverty, Race, and Public Health in the United States* (Baltimore, MD: Johns Hopkins University Press, 2001).

32. Safford, "De Soto's Descendant."

33. Nancy Rockafellar and James W. Haviland, "The Broad Sweep: A Chronological Summary of the First 100 Years of Medicine and Dentistry in Washington State, 1889–1989," in *Saddlebags to Scanners: The First 100 Years of Medicine in Washington State*, ed. Nancy Rockafellar and James W. Haviland (Seattle: Washington State Medical Association, Education and Research Foundation, 1989), 1–26.

34. Malcolm McDonald, "The Samaritan Spirit—Seattle's Pharisees," *Commonwealth*, May 23, 1903, 3.

35. Buerge, *Seattle in the 1880s*.

36. "Scenes in the Wayside Mission," 16.

37. "The Passion Play at the Jefferson Theater," *Seattle Post-Intelligencer*, June 25, 1899.

38. "Divine Healing Fails," *Seattle Post-Intelligencer*, July 3, 1899.

39. "Didn't Pray Hard Enough," *Evening Times*, July 6, 1899.

40. "Divine Healing Fails," 40.

41. Sally Sheard and Helen Power, "Body and the City: Medical and Urban Histories of Public Health," in *Body and City: Histories of Urban Public Health*, ed. Sally Sheard and Helen Power (Burlington, VT: Ashgate, 2000), 1–16.

42. Oscar R. Ewing, "History of the United States Public Health Service, 1798–1948," *Public Health News* 29, no. 9 (1948): 275–78.

43. Erika Janik, *Marketplace of the Marvelous: The Strange Origins of Modern Medicine* (Boston: Beacon, 2014); Jeremy Agnew, *Alcohol and Opium in the Old West: Use, Abuse, and Influence* (Jefferson, NC: McFarland, 2014).

44. Janik.

45. Gregg Olsen, *Starvation Heights: A True Story of Murder and Malice in the Woods of the Pacific Northwest* (1997; repr., New York: Three Rivers, 2005).

46. Kathrine Beck, "Hazzard, Linda Burfield (1867–1938)," *HistoryLink*, October 26, 2006, https://www.historylink.org/File/7955.

47. "The Doctor Who Starved Her Patients to Death," *Smithsonian*, October 28, 2014, https://www.smithsonianmag.com/history/doctor-who-starved-her-patients-death-180953158/.

48. "Twenty Men Locked in Wayside Mission Quarantined by Health Officer," *Seattle Post-Intelligencer*, July 12, 1899.

49. Kenneth L. Kusmer, *Down and Out, on the Road: The Homeless in American History*, rev. ed. (Oxford: Oxford University Press, 2003).

50. Todd DePastino, *Citizen Hobo: How a Century of Homelessness Shaped America* (Chicago: University of Chicago Press, 2003).

51. DePastino, 8.

52. Tim Cresswell, *The Tramp in America* (London: Reaktion, 2001).

53. Jack London, *Jack London on the Road: The Tramp Diary, and Other Hobo Writings* (Logan: Utah State University Press, 1979).

54. London, 100.

55. "She Flooded Them Out," *Seattle Post-Intelligencer*, September 29, 1899.

56. "Mourners Say Mrs. Johnson Threw Cold Water on a Funeral," *Seattle Post-Intelligencer*, December 12, 1899.

57. "Mourners Say Mrs. Johnson Threw Cold Water," 6.

58. "Scenes in the Wayside Mission," 16.

59. Walter I. Trattner, *From Poor Law to Welfare State: A History of Social Welfare in America*, 6th ed. (New York: Free Press, 1999).

60. John Putman, "A 'Test of Chiffon Politics': Gender Politics in Seattle, 1897–1917," *Pacific Historical Review* 69, no. 4 (2000): 595–616, https://doi.org/10.2307/3641226.

61. White, *New History of the American West*, 311.

62. Mary T. Henry, "Atlantic Street Center (Seattle)," *HistoryLink*, December 18, 2010, https://www.historylink.org/File/9613.

63. Dale Edward Soden, *The Reverend Mark Matthews: An Activist in the Progressive Era* (Seattle: University of Washington Press, 2001).

64. Richard C. Berner, *Seattle, 1900–1920: From Boomtown, Urban Turbulence, to Restoration* (Seattle, WA: Charles Press, 2009).

65. Ragnar T. Westman, *History of Prostitution in Seattle* (Seattle, WA: Seattle Department of Health and Sanitation, 1943).

66. "Dr. De Soto and His Work," *Seattle Post-Intelligencer*, October 28, 1900.

67. King County Washington Commissioners, *Beginnings, Progress and Achievement in the Medical Work of King County, Washington* (Seattle, WA: Peters Publishing, 1930).

68. Alex[ander] de Soto and C. W. Crimpton, "Coughs and Their Treatment," *Medical Bulletin* (1903): 17–22.

69. Clarence Bagley, *History of King County, Washington* (Seattle, WA: Clarke Publishing, 1929), 14.

70. Clarence B. Bagley, *History of Seattle*, vol. 2 (Seattle, WA: Jazzybee Verlag, n.d.).

71. Katharine Major, "Nursing Seattle's Unfortunate Sick," *American Journal of Nursing* 6, no. 1 (1905): 32–34.

72. "Editorial Comment," *American Journal of Nursing* 6, no. 1 (1905): 5–8.

73. King County Washington Commissioners, *Beginnings, Progress and Achievement*.

74. "The Northland: The Latest News from Reliable Sources concerning the Great North, Condensed," *Douglas Island News* (Douglas City, AK), November 28, 1906, https://chroniclingamerica.loc.gov/lccn/sn84021930/1906-11-28/ed-1/seq-1/.

75. Alexander de Soto and Irene de Soto's marriage certificate, King County, series A, #27787, January 13, 1934, King County Archives, Seattle, WA.

76. "Dr. De Soto, 96, Dies after Falling into Bay," *Brooklyn Daily Eagle*, November 12, 1936.

CHAPTER 5. SHACKTOWN

1. Susan Starbuck, *Hazel Wolf: Fighting the Establishment* (Seattle: University of Washington Press, 2002), 9–10.

2. Starbuck.

3. Letter to Dave Brower, February 19, 1996, Hazel Wolf Papers, Correspondence, 3647.008, University of Washington, Special Collections.

4. Carlos A. Schwantes, *Radical Heritage: Labor, Socialism, and Reform in Washington and British Columbia, 1885–1917* (Seattle: University of Washington Press, 1979).

5. Starbuck, *Hazel Wolf*, 61.

6. Starbuck, 58.

7. Starbuck, 83.

8. Richard C. Berner, *Seattle, 1900–1920: From Boomtown, Urban Turbulence, to Restoration* (Seattle, WA: Charles Press, 2009).

9. Meridel Le Sueur, "Waiting Was the Worst Part," in *The Great Depression*, ed. Dennis Nishi (San Diego, CA: Greenhaven, 2001), 56–66, 63.

10. Starbuck, *Hazel Wolf*, 37–38.

11. David B. Williams, *Too High and Too Steep: Reshaping Seattle's Topography* (Seattle: University of Washington Press, 2015).

12. "Racial Restrictive Covenants," Seattle Civil Rights and Labor History Project, accessed August 20, 2019, https://depts.washington.edu/civilr/covenants.htm#north.

13. Richard C. Berner, *Seattle, 1921–1940: From Boom to Bust* (Seattle, WA: Charles Press, 1992), 183.

14. Matthew Klingle, "Changing Spaces: Nature, Property, and Power in Seattle, 1880–1945," *Journal of Urban History* 32, no. 2 (January 2006): 197–230, 209, https://doi.org/10.1177/0096144205281613.

15. Theodore Roosevelt Center, "Address by President Roosevelt before the National Congress of Mothers," March 13, 1905, https://www.theodorerooseveltcenter.org/Research/Digital-Library/Record?libID=0280100.

16. Starbuck, *Hazel Wolf*.

17. Dale Edward Soden, *The Reverend Mark Matthews: An Activist in the Progressive Era* (Seattle: University of Washington Press, 2001).

18. Marion Hathway and John Rademaker, *Public Relief in Washington, 1853–1933: Poor Relief, Mothers' Pensions, Indigent Soldiers' Relief, Old Age Pensions, and Indigent Blind Relief in Washington* (Olympia: State of Washington Emergency Relief Administration, 1934).

19. Brianne Cook, "*Watcher on the Tower* and the Washington State Ku Klux Klan," Seattle Civil Rights and Labor History Project, accessed August 17, 2019, https://depts.washington.edu/civilr/kkk_wot.htm.

20. Lorraine McConaghy, *New Land, North of the Columbia: Historic Documents That Tell the Story of Washington State from Territory to Today* (Seattle, WA: Sasquatch Books, 2011).

21. Paula Becker, "Federal Theatre Project," *HistoryLink*, October 30, 2002, https://www.historylink.org/File/3978.

22. Hazel Wolf, "The Long Perspective on Environmental Activism," YouTube, April 25, 2014, https://www.youtube.com/watch?v=9uxy1ZWZ_G4.

23. Sarah Guthu, "Living Newspapers: One-Third of the Nation" (2009), Civil Rights and Labor History Consortium, http://depts.washington.edu/depress/theater_arts_living_newspaper_onethird.shtml.

24. Barry Witham, *The Federal Theatre Project: A Case Study* (New York: Cambridge University Press, 2003); Guthu, "Living Newspapers."

25. Starbuck, *Hazel Wolf*, 258.

26. Barron H. Lerner, *Contagion and Confinement: Controlling Tuberculosis along the Skid Road* (Baltimore, MD: Johns Hopkins University Press, 1998), 5.

27. Monte Holm, *Once a Hobo: The Autobiography of Monte Holm* (Ann Arbor, MI: Proctor, 1999), 185.

28. Vance M. Ardeune to City Council, October 10, 1938, CF 160628, Comptroller Files, Seattle Municipal Archives.

29. Lisa Goff, *Shantytown, USA: Forgotten Landscapes of the Working Poor* (Cambridge, MA: Harvard University Press, 2016), 50.

30. Doris McIlroy, "Shacktown Boom Arouses Citizens," *Seattle Post-Intelligencer*, December 6, 1938, pt. 2, pg. 11.

31. Dustin Neighly, "'Nobody Paid Any Attention': The Economic Marginalization of Seattle's Hooverville," Civil Rights and Labor History Consortium, 2010, http://depts.washington.edu/depress/hooverville_seattle_destruction.shtml.

32. May Gamble Young to City Council, April 24, 1937, CF 154992, Comptroller Files, 1802-01, Seattle Municipal Archives.

33. "Exhibit C: Basic Data concerning Physical Conditions and Occupancy of Shacks," March 5, 1941, CF 16942, Comptroller Files, 1802-01, Seattle Municipal Archives.

34. Shack Elimination Committee to Public Safety Committee, April 14, 1941, CF 169237, Comptroller Files, 1802-01, Seattle Municipal Archives.

35. "Department of Health and Sanitation of the City of Seattle, Wash., Annual Report: 1932 to 1935," December 31, 1935, Health Department Annual Reports, 1802-G6, Seattle Municipal Archives.

36. Shack Elimination Committee to Public Safety Committee.

37. Neighly, "Nobody Paid Any Attention."

38. Starbuck, *Hazel Wolf*, 85.

39. Walter I. Trattner, *From Poor Law to Welfare State: A History of Social Welfare in America*, 6th ed. (New York: Free Press, 1999).

40. Michael B. Katz, *In the Shadow of the Poorhouse* (New York: Basic, 1986).

41. Alice Willard Solenberger, *One Thousand Homeless Men: A Study of Original Records* (New York: Charities Publication Committee, Russell Sage Foundation, 1911), http://babel.hathitrust.org/cgi/pt?id=uc2 .ark:/13960/t7fq9t97r; Nels Anderson, *The Hobo: The Sociology of the Homeless Man* (Chicago: University of Chicago Press, 1923).

42. Allen R. Potter, *Facilities for Housing, Medical Care, and Other Services for Homeless Men in Seattle 1929–30* (Seattle: Washington State Conference of Social Work with cooperation of Department of Sociology, University of Washington, and Seattle Community Fund, 1930), Allen R. Potter Papers, 1930–1987, University of Washington, Special Collections; Donald Francis Roy, "Hooverville: A Study of a Community of Homeless Men in Seattle," University of Washington, 1935.

43. Annette de Vol Trumbull, "The Story of Hooverville in Seattle," term paper, University of Washington, July 1, 1935, University of Washington, Special Collections.

44. Dean Stiff, *The Milk and Honey Route: A Handbook for Hobos* (New York: Vanguard, 1931), 144–45.

45. Clare Coss, ed., *Lillian D. Wald: Progressive Activist* (New York: Feminist Press at the City University of New York, 1989); Patricia

D'Antonio, *American Nursing: A History of Knowledge, Authority, and the Meaning of Work* (Baltimore, MD: Johns Hopkins University Press, 2010).

46. Katz, *In the Shadow of the Poorhouse*; B. Ehrenreich and D. English, *Witches, Midwives and Nurses: A History of Women Healers* (New York: Feminist Press, 2010).

47. Coss, *Lillian D. Wald*.

48. J. A. Kenney, "The National Health Act of 1939," *Journal of the National Medical Association* 31, no. 4 (1939): 154–60.

49. Gordon Black, "Organizing the Unemployed: The Early 1930s," Civil Rights and Labor History Consortium, accessed August 3, 2019, http://depts.washington.edu/labhist/cpproject/black.shtml.

50. Tillie Olsen, "Thousand Dollar Vagrant," in Olsen, *Tell Me a Riddle, Requa I, and Other Works* (Lincoln: University of Nebraska Press, 2013), 149–54.

51. Wolf, "Long Perspective on Environmental Activism."

52. "Introduction: Communism in Washington State," Civil Rights and Labor History Consortium, accessed December 25, 2019, https://depts.washington.edu/labhist/cpproject/.

53. Mary McCarthy, "Circus Politics in Washington State," *Nation* 143, no. 16 (October 17, 1936): 442–44.

54. Black, "Organizing the Unemployed," 5.

55. Soden, *Reverend Mark Matthews*, 131.

56. Norman H. Clark, *The Dry Years: Prohibition and Social Change in Washington* (Seattle: University of Washington Press, 1965).

57. Seattle–King County Department of Public Health, *Public Health Then and Now: 1889 to 1989* (Seattle: Seattle–King County Department of Public Health, 1989).

58. Calvin Fisher Schmid, *Social Trends in Seattle* (Seattle: University of Washington Press, 1944).

59. Markel, "Contagion and Confinement."

60. "Eugenics and Disability: History and Legacy in Washington," Disability Studies, College of Arts and Sciences, University of Washington, accessed August 20, 2019, https://disabilitystudies.washington.edu/eugenics-and-disability-history-and-legacy-washington.

61. Lutz Kaelber, "Washington Eugenics," University of Vermont, accessed August 20, 2019, http://www.uvm.edu/~lkaelber/eugenics/WA/WAold.html.

62. "Eugenics and Disability."

63. Harborview Medical Center, *Harborview Medical Center, 1877–1977: A Century of Community Service and Caring* (Seattle, WA: Harborview Medical Center, 1978).

64. Coll Thrush, "Hauntings as Histories: Indigenous Ghosts and the Urban Past in Seattle," in *Phantom Past, Indigenous Presence: Native Ghosts in North American Culture and History*, ed. Colleen E. Boyd and Coll Thrush (Lincoln: University of Nebraska Press, 2011), 54–81; Coll Thrush, *Native Seattle: Histories from the Crossing-Over Place*, 2nd ed. (Seattle: University of Washington Press, 2017).

65. Starbuck, *Hazel Wolf*.

66. Priscilla Long, curator, "Seattle's First Hill: King County Courthouse and Harborview Hospital," *HistoryLink*, March 22, 2001, https://www.historylink.org/File/7038.

67. King County Washington Commissioners, *Beginnings, Progress and Achievement in the Medical Work of King County, Washington* (Seattle, WA: Peters Publishing, 1930).

68. Klingle, "Changing Spaces," 209.

69. Berner, *Seattle, 1921–1940*.

70. Richard Rothstein, *The Color of Law: A Forgotten History of How Our Government Segregated America* (London: Liveright, 2017).

71. Irene Burns Miller, *Profanity Hill* (Everett, WA: Working Press, 1979).

72. Studs Terkel, "Hazel Wolf, 95," in Terkel, *Coming of Age: The Story of Our Century by Those Who've Lived It* (New York: New Press, 1995), 136–41.

73. John H. Cushman Jr., "Hazel Wolf, 101: Fought for the Environment," *New York Times*, January 24, 2000, https://www.nytimes.com/2000/01/24/us/hazel-wolf-101-fought-for-the-environment.html; Susan Starbuck, "Crossing Boundaries: Hazel Wolf inside the Environmental Establishment," *Pacific Northwest Quarterly* 96, no. 2 (2005): 85–94.

74. Hazel Wolf, "Environmental Justice Coalition-Building in Seattle," *Race, Poverty and the Environment* 4, no. 2 (1993): 44.

1. Cheryl McCall and Mary Ellen Mark, "Streets of the Lost: Runaway Kids Eke Out a Mean Life in Seattle," *Life*, July 1983, http://www.maryellenmark.com/text/magazines/life/905W-000-021.html.

2. Anne Focke, *Sustaining a Vital Downtown Community: A Study of the Market Foundation of Seattle* (Seattle, WA: Market Foundation, 1987).

3. Coll Thrush, *Native Seattle: Histories from the Crossing-Over Place*, 2nd ed. (Seattle: University of Washington Press, 2017); William C. Speidel, *Sons of the Profits: The Seattle Story, 1851–1901; or, There's No Business like Grow Business*, 2nd ed. (Seattle, WA: Nettle Creek, 1968).

4. "The New Frontier," acceptance speech of Senator John F. Kennedy, Democratic National Convention, July 15, 1960, John F. Kennedy Library, https://www.jfklibrary.org/asset-viewer/archives/JFKSEN/0910/JFKSEN-0910-015; Mark J. White, *Kennedy: The New Frontier Revisited* (New York: New York University Press, 1998).

5. Thrush, *Native Seattle*; Paula Becker, "Century 21 Exposition Official Ewen Dingwall Closes Controversial 'Girls of the Galaxy' Show on May 13, 1962," *HistoryLink*, February 16, 2011, https://www.historylink.org/File/10008.

6. Greg Lange, "President Kennedy Delivers Major Policy Speech at UW on November 16, 1961," *HistoryLink*, March 16, 1999, https://www.historylink.org/File/968.

7. Murray Morgan, *Skid Road: An Informal Portrait of Seattle*, 2nd ed. (1982; repr., Seattle: University of Washington Press, 2018), 65.

8. Roger Conant, *Mercer's Belles: The Journal of a Reporter* (Seattle: University of Washington Press, 1960).

9. Conant.

10. Alan J. Stein, "*Here Come the Brides* Debuts on ABC on September 25, 1968," *HistoryLink*, November 19, 2018, https://historylink.org/file/1563.

11. "President Kennedy Delivers Major Policy Speech."

12. Thrush, *Native Seattle*; Sinan Demirel, "Homeless in Seattle: The Roots of a Crisis,"*Crosscut*, July 26, 2016, http://features.crosscut.com/homeless-in-seattle-the-roots-of-a-crisis.

13. Knute Berger, "How Seattle Stopped a Freeway, and May Gain a Monument," *Crosscut*, October 6, 2016, https://crosscut.com/2016/10/how-seattle-stopped-a-freeway-and-may-gain-a-monument; Knute

Berger, "Remembering Seattle's Anti-Freeway Crusaders," *Seattle Magazine*, November 27, 2018, https://www.seattlemag.com/news-and -features/remembering-seattle-anti-freeway-crusaders.

14. National League of Cities—United States Conference of Mayors, Center for Policy Analysis, *The Mayor and Model Cities* (Washington, DC: National League of Cities and the US Conference of Mayors, 1971).

15. Keith B. Vaughan and Lee G. Copeland, *Seattle Model City Housing and Physical Environment Program Evaluation* (Seattle, WA: Seattle Model City Program, 1971), 50.

16. National League of Cities—United States Conference of Mayors, *The Mayor and Model Cities*; Seattle Model City Program, *City of Seattle Model Cities Program* (Seattle, WA: n.p., 1968).

17. Vaughan and Copeland, *Seattle Model City Housing*, 2.

18. Jim Kershner, "Boeing and Washington's Aerospace Industry, 1934–2015," *HistoryLink*, September 8, 2015, https://www.historylink. org/File/11111.

19. Greg Lange, "Billboard Reading 'Will the Last Person Leaving SEATTLE—Turn Out the Lights' Appears near Sea-Tac International Airport on April 16, 1971," *HistoryLink*, June 8, 1999, https://www .historylink.org/File/1287.

20. Laurie Olin, *Breath on the Mirror: Seattle's Skid Road Community* (Seattle, WA: Laurie Olin, 1972).

21. Laurie Olin, "From Sundogs to the Midnight Sun: An Alaskan Reverie," *Hudson Review* 66, no. 1 (2013): 50–93.

22. Olin, *Breath on the Mirror*, 28.

23. Kim Hopper and Jill Hamberg, *The Making of America's Homeless from Skid Row to New Poor, 1945–1984* (New York: Community Service Society of New York, 1984), 13.

24. E. Fuller Torrey, *American Psychosis: How the Federal Government Destroyed the Mental Illness Treatment System* (Oxford: Oxford University Press, 2014).

25. Ken Kesey, *One Flew over the Cuckoo's Nest* (New York: Signet, 1962).

26. Mary Ellen Mark, *Ward 81* (1979; repr., Bologna, Italy: Damiani, 2008).

27. Torrey, *American Psychosis*.

28. Torrey.

29. Torrey.

30. Torrey.

31. Ron Judd, "An Old Mental Institution, and Its Cemetery, Might Get a Dignified Makeover," *Seattle Times*, April 6, 2017, https://www.seattletimes.com/pacific-nw-magazine/an-old-mental-institution-and-its-cemetery-might-get-a-dignified-makeover/.

32. Chris Wedes, *J. P. Patches, Northwest Icon* (Seattle, WA: Peanut Butter Publishers, 2002).

33. Tim Cresswell, *The Tramp in America* (London: Reaktion, 2001).

34. Joe Martin, Skid Road Oral History, interview by author, May 4, 2017.

35. Charles Royer, Skid Road Oral History, interview by author, June 21, 2017.

36. Joel L. Fleishman, *The Foundation: A Great American Secret: How Private Wealth Is Changing the World* (New York: Public Affairs, 2007).

37. Philip W. Brickner, *Health Care of Homeless People* (New York: Springer, 1985).

38. Josephine Ensign, *Health Care for the Homeless: A Vision of Health for All* (Nashville, TN: National Health Care for the Homeless Council, August 30, 2016).

39. Brickner, *Health Care of Homeless People.*

40. Ron Ruthruff, *The Least of These: Lessons Learned from Kids on the Street* (Birmingham, AL: New Hope, 2011).

41. Sinan Demirel, "When We Paid Caseworkers in Cookies: A Brief History of Serving Homeless Youth," *Crosscut*, March 4, 2014, https://crosscut.com/2014/03/history-homeless-youth-services-king-county-demire.

42. Jack Kerouac, *Desolation Angels* (1965; repr., New York: Riverhead, 1995), 123.

43. Knute Berger, "Seattle's Creepy Donut Shop: The Inside Story," March 19, 2014, https://crosscut.com/2014/03/seattle-donut-shop-runaways-part-two-knute-berger.

44. Jim Theofelis, Skid Road Oral History, interview by author, October 22, 2015.

45. Theofelis interview.

46. Justin Reed Early, *Streetchild: An Unpaved Passage* (Bloomington, IN: AuthorHouse, 2008), 21.

47. Mary Ellen Mark, *Tiny: Streetwise Revisited* (New York: Aperture, 2015).

48. Mary Ellen Mark, *Streetwise* (Philadelphia: University of Pennsylvania Press, 1988), 61.

49. Mark, *Streetwise*, 66.

50. McCall and Mark, "Streets of the Lost."

51. Carol Ostrom, "Street Life Is Grim for Teen-Age Runaways," *Seattle Times*, December 5, 1982, A-1.

52. Ostrom.

53. Ostrom.

54. "A Red Light History of Seattle," *Seattle Met*, February 2010, https://www.seattlemet.com/articles/2010/1/29/red-light-history-0210.

55. Kaiser Family Foundation, "Medicare and Medicaid at 50," YouTube, April 21, 2015, https://www.youtube.com/watch?v=f9NUCvrrRz4.

56. David E. Smith et al., eds., *The Free Clinic: A Community Approach to Health Care and Drug Abuse* (Beloit, WI: Stash Press, 1971).

57. Gregory L. Weiss, *Grassroots Medicine: The Story of America's Free Health Clinics* (Lanham, MD: Rowman and Littlefield, 2006).

58. Smith et al., *Free Clinic*.

59. Mavis Bonnar, Skid Road Oral History, interview by author, March 6, 2017.

60. Lee Kirschner, "Delivery of Service through a Grass Roots Community Agency," 1969, Open Door Clinic, University of Washington, Special Collections.

61. Weiss, *Grassroots Medicine*.

62. Jim McDermott, Skid Road Oral History, interview by author, October 28, 2016.

63. David Wilma, "Amphetamines Constitute Largest Drug Problem in Seattle's University District as of January 7, 1968," *HistoryLink*, May 24, 2001, https://www.historylink.org/File/3306.

64. Martin interview.

65. Bonnar interview.

66. Robert Deisher, Greg Robinson, and Debra Boyer, "The Adolescent Female and Male Prostitute," *Pediatric Annals* 11, no. 10 (1982): 819–25, https://doi.org/10.3928/0090-4481-19821001-10; R. W. Deisher, V. Eisner, and S. I. Sulzbacher, "The Young Male Prostitute," *Pediatrics* 43, no. 6 (1969): 936–41; Robert Deisher and James Farrow, "Recognizing and Dealing with Alienated Youth in Clinical Practice," *Pediatric Annals* 15, no. 11 (1986): 759–64, https://doi.org/10.3928/0090-4481-19861101-05.

67. McCall and Mark, "Streets of the Lost."

68. Mary Ellen Mark, *On the Portrait and the Moment* (New York: Aperture, 2015).

69. Mark, 74, 68.

70. Evan Louison, "The Full-Time Job of Survival: Martin Bell on *Streetwise* and *Tiny: The Life of Erin Blackwell*," *Filmmaker Magazine*, June 23, 2016, https://filmmakermagazine.com/98908-full-time-job-of -survival-martin-bell-on-streetwise-and-tiny-the-life-of-erin-blackwell/.

71. Mark, *On the Portrait and the Moment*, 83.

72. Early, *Streetchild*.

73. Early.

74. Caden Mark Gardner, "Why We Never Forgot Tiny," *Metrograph*, July 17, 2019, http://metrograph.com/edition/article/107/why-we -never-forgot-tiny.

75. Mark, *Tiny*, 48.

76. Mueblespasayo, "Lost Seattle: The Monastery Chronicles," *Cloud Transit*, August 2, 2015, https://cloudtransit.wordpress.com/2015/08/02/ lost-seattle-the-monastery-chronicles/.

77. Ben Jacklet, "The Return of the Demon," *Stranger*, September 2, 1999, https://www.thestranger.com/seattle/the-return-of-the-demon/ Content?oid=1895.

78. Alison G. Ivey, "Washington's Becca Bill: The Costs of Empowering Parents," *Seattle University Law Review* 20, no. 1 (1996): 125–56.

79. Tiffany Zwicker Eggers, "The Becca Bill Would Not Have Saved Becca: Washington State's Treatment of Young Female Offenders," *Law and Inequality: A Journal of Theory and Practice* 16, no. 1 (n.d.): 219–58.

80. Theofelis interview.

81. Early, *Streetchild*, xii.

82. Mark, *Tiny*, 73.

83. Nicole Brodeur, "Three Decades after 'Streetwise' Documentary, 'Tiny' Struggles and Dreams On," *Seattle Times*, May 20, 2016, https:// www.seattletimes.com/entertainment/movies/three-decades-after- streetwise-documentary-tiny-struggles-and-dreams-on/.

84. Khadija Diallo, "The Fight for Her Life—'Streetwise' and Keanna's Triumphant Story," Project on Family Homelessness, October 21, 2016, https://projectonfamilyhomelessness.org/2016/10/21/the-fight-for-her -life-streetwise-and-keannas-triumphant-story/.

85. Mark, *Tiny*, 5.

86. Brodeur, "Three Decades after 'Streetwise' Documentary."

87. Nicola Slawson, "Can the Mockingbird Model of Foster Care Fly in the UK?" *Guardian*, April 28, 2016, https://www.theguardian.com/social -care-network/2016/apr/28/mockingbird-foster-care-uk-social-work.

88. Anne K. Ream, "The Advocate: Noel Gomez," World without Exploitation, accessed October 29, 2019, https://www .worldwithoutexploitation.org/survivor/noel-gomez.

CHAPTER 7. STATE OF EMERGENCY

1. Walt Crowley, "Earthquake Registering 6.8 on Richter Scale Jolts Seattle and Puget Sound on February 28, 2001," *HistoryLink*, March 1, 2001, https://historylink.org/File/3039; Rob Harrill, "Damaged Chimneys and Unexpected Liquefaction from Nisqually Temblor Yield Earthquake Insights, UW Scientists Say," *UW News*, April 17, 2001, https://www.washington.edu/news/2001/04/17/damaged-chimneys -and-unexpected-liquefaction-from-nisqually-temblor-yield-earthquake -insights-uw-scientists-say/.

2. Alex Fryer, "Earthquake Windfall Goes to the Homeless," *Seattle Times*, May 28, 2001, http://community.seattletimes.nwsource.com/ archive/?date=20010528&slug=bigcheck28m.

3. Scott Greenstone, "You're Homeless, but You Have to Leave the Hospital: Where Do You Go?," *Seattle Times*, December 24, 2018, https:// www.seattletimes.com/seattle-news/homeless/sick-homeless-people -get-stuck-in-washington-hospitals-but-theres-a-solution/.

4. Rebecca Hersher and Robert Benincasa, "How Federal Disaster Money Favors the Rich," NPR, March 5, 2019, https://www.npr.org/ 2019/03/05/688786177/how-federal-disaster-money-favors-the-rich.

5. Office of the Mayor, "Murray, Constantine, City Council Declare Emergency, Announce New Investments to Respond to Homelessness," November 2, 2015, http://murray.seattle.gov/murray-constantine-city -council-declare-emergency-announce-new-investments-to-respond -to-homelessness/; "King County Homelessness Emergency Response," accessed November 18, 2019, https://www.kingcounty.gov/depts/ community-human-services/housing/services/homeless-housing/ kc-hmlsns-resp.aspx.

6. Margot Kushel, "Why There Are So Many Unsheltered Home-

less People on the West Coast," *Conversation*, accessed November 24, 2019, http://theconversation.com/why-there-are-so-many-unsheltered -homeless-people-on-the-west-coast-96767.

7. Peter Bergman et al., "Creating Moves to Opportunity," Opportunity Insights, August 2019, https://opportunityinsights.org/paper/ cmto/.

8. Nicholas Kristof, "A Better Address Can Change a Child's Future," *New York Times*, August 3, 2019, https://www.nytimes.com/2019/08/03/ opinion/sunday/poverty-seattle.html; Bergman et al., "Creating Moves to Opportunity."

9. "Support for First-Time Moms," Nurse-Family Partnership, accessed December 7, 2019, https://www.nursefamilypartnership.org/ first-time-moms/; Katherine Boo, "Swamp Nurse," *New Yorker*, January 30, 2006, https://www.newyorker.com/magazine/2006/02/06/swamp -nurse.

10. Elizabeth Kneebone, "The Changing Geography of US Poverty," Brookings Institution, February 15, 2017, https://www.brookings.edu/ testimonies/the-changing-geography-of-us-poverty/.

11. Benjamin Danielson, Skid Road Oral History, interview by author, November 2, 2015.

12. Danielson interview.

13. Nancy Sugg, Skid Road Oral History, interview by author, March 10, 2017.

14. Seattle Housing and and Resource Effort / Women's Housing Equality and Enhancement League, accessed December 15, 2019, http:// www.sharewheel.org/.

15. Josh Cohen, "King County Lost FEMA Homelessness Funding Because the Region Is Too Wealthy," *Crosscut*, August 30, 2019, https:// crosscut.com/2019/08/king-county-lost-fema-homelessness-funding -because-region-too-wealthy.

16. Jim Theofelis, Skid Road Oral History, interview by author, October 22, 2015.

17. Theofelis interview.

18. A Way Home Washington, "Prevent and End Youth Homelessness," accessed December 15, 2019, https://awayhomewa.org/.

19. Sinan Demirel, Skid Road Oral History, interview by author, February 23, 2017.

20. Drew Atkins, "The Man Who Tried to End Homelessness," *Cross-

cut, July 5, 2016, https://crosscut.com/2016/07/the-man-who-tried-to
-end-homelessness.

21. Steve Berg, "Ten-Year Plans to End Homelessness," National Low
Income Housing Coalition, *2015 Advocates' Guide*, 26–27, https://nlihc
.org/sites/default/files/Sec7.08_Ten-Year-Plan_2015.pdf.

22. Ella Howard, *Homeless: Poverty and Place in Urban America* (Philadelphia: University of Pennsylvania Press, 2013); Jason Adam Was-
serman, *At Home on the Street: People, Poverty, and a Hidden Culture of
Homelessness* (Boulder, CO: Lynne Rienner, 2010); Craig Willse, *The Value
of Homelessness: Managing Surplus Life in the United States* (Minneapolis:
University of Minnesota Press, 2015).

23. Deborah Padgett, *Housing First: Ending Homelessness, Transforming
Systems, and Changing Lives* (New York: Oxford University Press, 2016).

24. Josephine Ensign, *Health Care for the Homeless: A Vision of Health
for All* (Nashville, TN: National Health Care for the Homeless Council,
August 30, 2016).

25. Samantha Artiga and Elizabeth Hinton, "Beyond Health Care:
The Role of Social Determinants in Promoting Health and Health Equity," Kaiser Family Foundation, May 10, 2018, https://www.kff.org/
disparities-policy/issue-brief/beyond-health-care-the-role-of-social
-determinants-in-promoting-health-and-health-equity/.

26. Erica C. Barnett, "After 15 Years, Seattle's Radical Experiment in
No-Barrier Housing Is Still Saving Lives," *Crosscut*, accessed September
25, 2019, https://crosscut.com/2019/09/after-15-years-seattles-radical
-experiment-no-barrier-housing-still-saving-lives.

27. Mary E. Larimer et al., "Health Care and Public Service Use and
Costs before and after Provision of Housing for Chronically Homeless Persons with Severe Alcohol Problems," *JAMA* 301, no. 13 (April 1,
2009): 1349–57, https://doi.org/10.1001/jama.2009.414; Bonnie Burl-
ingham et al., "A House Is Not a Home: A Qualitative Assessment of the
Life Experiences of Alcoholic Homeless Women," *Journal of Social Work
Practice in the Addictions* 10, no. 2 (May 25, 2010): 158–79, https://doi
.org/10.1080/15332561003741921; Susan E. Collins et al., "Project-Based
Housing First for Chronically Homeless Individuals with Alcohol Problems: Within-Subjects Analyses of 2-Year Alcohol Trajectories," *American
Journal of Public Health* 102, no. 3 (2012): 511–19, https://doi.org/10.2105/
AJPH.2011.300403.

28. Barnett, "After 15 Years, Seattle's Radical Experiment," 15.

29. Patt Morrison, "Original 'Skid Road': Homeless Add a Sad Note to Gentrified Seattle Area," *Los Angeles Times*, March 24, 1987, http://articles.latimes.com/1987-03-24/news/mn-299_1_skid-row.

30. Tony Sparks, "Governing the Homeless in an Age of Compassion: Homelessness, Citizenship, and the 10-Year Plan to End Homelessness in King County Washington," *Antipode* 44, no. 4 (2012): 1510–31, https://doi.org/10.1111/j.1467-8330.2011.00957.x.

31. Charissa Fotinos, Skid Road Oral History, interview by author, January 15, 2016.

32. Mark Putnam, Skid Road Oral History, interview by author, October 26, 2015.

33. Putnam interview; John Ryan, "After 10-Year Plan, Why Does Seattle Have More Homeless than Ever?," KUOW, March 3, 2015, http://archive.kuow.org/post/after-10-year-plan-why-does-seattle-have-more-homeless-ever.

34. "Redevelopment of Yesler Terrace," Seattle Housing Authority, accessed November 18, 2019, https://www.seattlehousing.org/about-us/redevelopment/redevelopment-of-yesler-terrace.

35. Daniel Beekman, "Seattle's New Yesler Terrace Park Opens in Heart of Mixed-Income Redevelopment," *Seattle Times*, August 31, 2018, https://www.seattletimes.com/seattle-news/politics/seattles-new-yesler-terrace-park-opens-at-heart-of-mixed-income-redevelopment/.

36. Vernal Coleman, "A New Way to Help Seattle's Homeless: Navigation Center Set to Open Wednesday," *Seattle Times*, July 10, 2017, https://www.seattletimes.com/seattle-news/northwest/navigation-center-for-seattle-homeless-to-open-next-week/.

37. Mike Baker, "Homeless Residents Got One-Way Tickets Out of Town: Many Returned to the Streets," *New York Times*, September 14, 2019, https://www.nytimes.com/2019/09/14/us/homeless-busing-seattle-san-francisco.html; Sydney Brownstone, "King County Council Will More than Triple the Funding to Reunite Homeless People with Their Families: It's Not Clear How Well It Will Work," *Seattle Times*, November 23, 2019, https://www.seattletimes.com/seattle-news/homeless/county-votes-to-more-than-triple-the-funding-available-to-reunite-homeless-people-with-their-families-its-not-clear-how-well-it-will-work/.

38. Brownstone, "King County Council Will More than Triple the Funding."

39. "Count Us In," All Home King County, accessed December 15, 2019, http://allhomekc.org/king-county-point-in-time-pit-count/.

40. Baker, "Homeless Residents Got One-Way Tickets."

41. Jay Willis, "Sweeps Trample the Rights and Lives of the City's Homeless," *Seattle Times*, May 24, 2016, https://www.seattletimes.com/opinion/sweeps-trample-the-rights-and-lives-of-the-citys-homeless/.

42. Timothy A. Gibson, *Securing the Spectacular City: The Politics of Revitalization and Homelessness in Downtown Seattle* (Lanham, MD: Lexington, 2004), 162.

43. Rick Reynolds, Skid Road Oral History, interview by author, March 6, 2017.

44. Gibson, *Securing the Spectacular City*.

45. Kirk Johnson, "Seattle Underbelly Exposed as Homeless Camp Violence Flares," *New York Times*, March 1, 2016, https://www.nytimes.com/2016/03/02/us/seattle-homeless-jungle-camp.html; Michael Miller, "Slaying in 'the Jungle': Deadly Shooting at Seattle Homeless Camp Deepens Crisis," *Washington Post*, January 27, 2016, https://www.washingtonpost.com/news/morning-mix/wp/2016/01/27/murder-in-the-jungle-deadly-shooting-at-seattle-homeless-camp-deepens-crisis/.

46. Frederick Jackson Turner, *The Frontier in American History* (New York: Holt, 1920), https://archive.org/details/frontierinamericooturnuoft/page/n4/mode/2up.

47. John M. Findlay, "Closing the Frontier in Washington: Edmond S. Meany and Frederick Jackson Turner," *Pacific Northwest Quarterly* 82, no. 2 (1991): 59–70, 65.

48. Findlay, 67.

49. Carl Abbott, *The Metropolitan Frontier: Cities in the Modern American West* (Tucson: University of Arizona Press, 1993).

50. Benjamin Wallace-Wells, "How the Minimum-Wage Movement Entered the Mainstream," *New Yorker*, March 31, 2016, https://www.newyorker.com/news/benjamin-wallace-wells/how-the-minimum-wage-movement-entered-the-mainstream.

51. Reynolds interview.

52. Ken Kraybill and Sharon Morrison, "Assessing Health, Promoting Wellness: Motivational Interviewing," *Homeless Hub*, 2011, https://www.homelesshub.ca/resource/assessing-health-promoting-wellness-motivational-interviewing; William Richard Miller and Stephen Roll-

nick, *Motivational Interviewing: Helping People Change*, 3rd ed. (New York: Guilford, 2013).

53. "Motivational Interviewing: A Collaborative Path to Change," *American Nurse*, March 11, 2011, https://www.americannursetoday.com/motivational-interviewing-a-collaborative-path-to-change/.

54. Ken Kraybill, Skid Road Oral History, interview by author, January 19, 2016.

55. Heather Barr, Skid Road Oral History, interview by author, October 27, 2015.

56. Barr interview.

57. Sara Jean Green, "'Buyer Beware': Early Success for Initiative Targeting Johns instead of Prostitutes," *Seattle Times*, May 16, 2015, https://www.seattletimes.com/seattle-news/crime/buyer-beware-early-success-for-initiative-targeting-johns-instead-of-prostitutes/.

58. James Stevens, "The Natural History of Seattle," *American Mercury* (December 1932): 402–9, 406.

59. Lynn Thompson, "Busted: How Police Brought Down a Tech-Savvy Prostitution Network in Bellevue," *Seattle Times*, July 26, 2017, http://projects.seattletimes.com/2017/eastside-prostitution-bust/.

60. Evan Bush, "New Report Highlights Flaws in Police Data on Missing, Murdered Indigenous Women and Girls," *Seattle Times*, November 14, 2018, https://www.seattletimes.com/seattle-news/new-report-highlights-flaws-in-police-data-on-missing-murdered-indigenous-women-and-girls/.

61. "Our Bodies, Our Stories," Urban Indian Health Institute, accessed December 15, 2019, https://www.uihi.org/projects/our-bodies-our-stories/.

62. Lauren Frohne and Bettina Hansen, "Not Invisible: Confronting a Crisis of Violence against Native Women," *Seattle Times*, August 11, 2019, https://projects.seattletimes.com/2019/mmiw/.

63. Krystal Koop, Skid Road Oral History, interview by author, July 1, 2015.

64. Koop interview.

65. Sara Jean Green, "'Still a Huge Wound': Remembering Green River Killer's Victims," *Seattle Times*, March 19, 2013, https://www.seattletimes.com/seattle-news/lsquostill-a-huge-woundrsquo-remembering-green-river-killerrsquos-victims/.

66. David Kroman, "With Alternatives Stretched and Neighbors

Angry, Seattle Police Return to Arresting Sex Workers," *Crosscut*, October 2, 2019, https://crosscut.com/2019/10/alternatives-stretched-and -neighbors-angry-seattle-police-return-arresting-sex-workers.

67. Rick Anderson, "Seattle Judge Rules a Homeless Man's Truck Was His 'Home,' and That Has City Officials Worried," *Los Angeles Times*, March 10, 2018, https://www.latimes.com/nation/la-na-seattle -homeless-20180310-story.html.

68. Hazel Wolf, "Environmental Justice Coalition-Building in Seattle," *Race, Poverty and the Environment* 4, no. 2 (1993): 44.

69. Lewis Kamb, "Police Officer Sues Seattle, Claiming Toxic Chemicals from Homeless-Camp Cleanup Sickened Him," *Seattle Times*, January 9, 2020, https://www.seattletimes.com/seattle-news/police -officer-sues-seattle-claiming-toxic-chemicals-from-homeless-camp -cleanup-sickened-him/.

70. Agency for Toxic Substances and Disease Registry, "Tox FAQs for Polychlorinated Biphenyls (PCBs)," July 2014, https://www.atsdr.cdc .gov/phs/phs.asp?id=140&tid=26.

71. Demirel interview.

72. Marc Stiles and Coral Garnick, "The Price of Homelessness: The Seattle Area Spends More than $1 Billion a Year on This Humanitarian Crisis," *Puget Sound Business Journal*, November 16, 2017, https:// www.bizjournals.com/seattle/news/2017/11/16/price-of-homelessness -seattle-king-county-costs.html.

73. Sharon Lee, "Tiny House Villages in Seattle: An Efficient Response to Our Homelessness Crisis," *Shelterforce*, March 15, 2019, https:// shelterforce.org/2019/03/15/tiny-house-villages-in-seattle-an-efficient -response-to-our-homelessness-crisis/.

74. Scott Greenstone, "Seven Months Ago, Residents Locked the City Out of Their Tiny House Village: Now, Seattle Officials Plan to Cut Its Funding," *Seattle Times*, October 29, 2019, https://www.seattletimes .com/seattle-news/homeless/seven-months-ago-residents-locked-the -city-out-of-their-tiny-house-village-now-seattle-officials-plan-to-cut-its -funding/.

75. Scott Greenstone, "Nickelsville Will Stay in Northlake Tiny Village until June: City Agrees, Citing Coronavirus," *Seattle Times*, March 18, 2020, https://www.seattletimes.com/seattle-news/homeless/ nickelsville-will-stay-in-northlake-tiny-house-village-until-june-city -agrees-citing-coronavirus/.

76. Stiles and Garnick, "The Price of Homelessness."

77. Maddy Reinert, Theresa Nguyen, and Danielle Fritze, "The State of Mental Health in America, 2020," Mental Health America, 2019, https://www.mhanational.org/sites/default/files/State%20of%20Mental%20Health%20in%20America%20-%202020.pdf.

78. Joseph O'Sullivan, "Western State Hospital Loses $53 Million in Federal Funding after Failing Inspection," *Seattle Times*, June 25, 2018, https://www.seattletimes.com/seattle-news/politics/western-state-hospital-loses-federal-funding-after-failing-inspection/.

79. Alana Semuels, "How Amazon Helped Kill a Seattle Tax on Business," *Atlantic*, June 13, 2018, https://www.theatlantic.com/technology/archive/2018/06/how-amazon-helped-kill-a-seattle-tax-on-business/562736/.

80. Robert Wynne, "Reaction to the Chinese in the Pacific Northwest and British Columbia, 1850 to 1910," PhD diss., University of Washington, 1964 (ProQuest).

81. "Ballard Man Defends Tactic to Counteract Homelessness after Finding Corpse," *MyNorthwest*, February 3, 2016, https://mynorthwest.com/170221/ballard-man-defends-tactic-to-counteract-homelessness-after-finding-corpse/.

82. "Ballard Town Hall Turns into an Angry Shoutfest," *My Ballard*, May 3, 2018, https://www.myballard.com/2018/05/03/ballard-town-hall-turns-into-an-angry-shoutfest/.

83. Eric Johnson, *Seattle Is Dying*, KOMO, March 14, 2019, https://komonews.com/news/local/komo-news-special-seattle-is-dying.

84. Johnson.

85. Johnson.

86. Roger Valdez, "Seattle Isn't Dying Yet, but the Latest Debate Might Kill It," *Forbes*, April 8, 2019, https://www.forbes.com/sites/rogervaldez/2019/04/08/seattle-isnt-dying-yet-but-the-latest-debate-might-kill-it/.

87. Ashley Archibald, "No: Seattle Isn't Dying," *Real Change*, November 6, 2019, https://www.realchangenews.org/2019/11/06/no-seattle-isnt-dying.

88. Catherine Hinrichsen, "6 Reasons Why KOMO's Take on Homelessness Is the Wrong One," *Crosscut*, March 20, 2019, https://crosscut.com/2019/03/6-reasons-why-komos-take-homelessness-wrong-one.

89. Anderson Cooper, "'Rent Is Obscene Here': The Issues Forcing People in Seattle onto the Street," *60 Minutes*, CBS, December 1, 2019, https://www.cbsnews.com/news/homeless-in-america-the-issues-forcing-people-in-seattle-onto-the-street-60-minutes-2019-12-01/.

90. Hannah Knowles, "Amazon Spent $1.5 Million on Seattle City Council Races: The Socialist It Opposed Has Won," *Washington Post*, November 10, 2019, https://www.washingtonpost.com/nation/2019/11/10/amazon-spent-million-seattle-city-council-races-socialist-it-opposed-has-won/.

91. Asia Fields, "'It Should Have Been Open a Year Ago': Homeless Shelter to Open in Seattle's Harborview Hall—but It Hasn't Been Easy," *Seattle Times*, July 30, 2018, https://www.seattletimes.com/seattle-news/homeless/two-years-later-homeless-shelter-in-seattles-harborview-hall-expected-to-open-in-fall/.

92. Audrey Young, *The House of Hope and Fear: Life in a Big City Hospital* (Seattle, WA: Sasquatch Books, 2010).

93. Linzi Sheldon, "King County: Use Empty Harborview Nurses' Dorm for Homeless Shelter," KIRO, November 21, 2016, http://www.kiro7.com/news/local/king-county-use-empty-harborview-nurses-dorm-for-homeless-shelter/469129568; King County, "Harborview Hall," accessed February 2, 2017, http://www.kingcounty.gov/services/home-property/historic-preservation/projects/harborview-hall.aspx; King County, "Harborview Hall Opening to Welcome Up to 100 Adults and Their Pets to Warm, Safe Shelter on First Hill," December 20, 2018, https://www.kingcounty.gov/elected/executive/constantine/news/release/2018/December/20-harborview-shelter.aspx.

94. King County, "King County Joins with Harborview Medical Center to Open COVID-19 Recovery Site," March 21, 2020, https://www.kingcounty.gov/elected/executive/constantine/news/release/2020/March/21-harborview-recovery-site.aspx.

95. Michael Copass, Skid Road Oral History, interview by author, July 26, 2015.

96. David Carlbom, Skid Road Oral History, interview by author, October 28, 2015.

97. Edward P. Weber, D. Denise Lach, and Brent Steel, *New Strategies for Wicked Problems: Science and Solutions in the Twenty-First Century* (Corvallis: Oregon State University Press, 2017), 2.

98. Weber, Lach, and Steel, 28.

99. Donald A. Schon, "The New Scholarship Requires a New Epistemology," *Change* 27, no. 6 (1995): 27–34, 27.

100. Schon, 28.

101. King County, "One Table: A Community Approach to Homelessness and Affordability," accessed November 16, 2019, https://www.kingcounty.gov/depts/community-human-services/housing/services/homeless-housing/one-table.aspx.

102. King County.

103. Murray Morgan, *Skid Road: An Informal Portrait of Seattle*, 2nd ed. (1982; repr., Seattle: University of Washington Press, 2018), 295.

104. Morgan, 294.

EPILOGUE. HEARING VOICES

1. Erik Lacitis, "The Solitary Life and Death of a Homeless Man and His Dog near the 520 Bridge," *Seattle Times*, August 25, 2019, https://www.seattletimes.com/seattle-news/hardly-a-ripple-the-solitary-life-and-death-of-a-homeless-man-near-the-520-bridge/.

2. Erik Lacitis, "Man Makes a Rowboat His Home under the 520 Bridge," *Seattle Times*, April 24, 2011, https://www.seattletimes.com/seattle-news/man-makes-a-rowboat-his-home-under-the-520-bridge/.

3. Scott Greenstone, "More Seattleites Are Housing Homeless People in Their Backyards, but It's Hard to Find the Right Fit," *Seattle Times*, November 18, 2019, https://www.seattletimes.com/seattle-news/homeless/more-seattleites-are-housing-homeless-people-in-their-backyards-but-its-happening-slowly/.

4. Craig Rennebohm, *Souls in the Hands of a Tender God: Stories of the Search for Home and Healing on the Streets* (Boston: Beacon, 2008).

5. Craig Rennebohm, Skid Road Oral History, interview by author, February 2, 2016.

6. Scott Greenstone, "A Cafe where No One Is Homeless: One Solution to Youth on Seattle Streets," *Seattle Times*, December 11, 2017, https://www.seattletimes.com/seattle-news/a-cafe-where-no-one-is-homeless-one-solution-to-youth-on-the-streets/.

7. Nancy Amidei, Skid Road Oral History, interview by author, June 16, 2015.

8. David Hitchcock (@Hitchcockian), Twitter, November 29, 2019, https://twitter.com/Hitchcockian/status/1200398866190929920.

9. Claudia Castro Luna, "Seattle's Poem," in Luna, *This City* (Seattle, WA: Floating Bridge Press, 2016), 27–29.

10. Coll Thrush, *Native Seattle: Histories from the Crossing-Over Place*, 2nd ed. (Seattle: University of Washington Press, 2017), 207.

INDEX

Louisville (Seattle shacktown), 126
Low Income Housing Institute, 216
LSD, 168, 176
Luna, Claudia Castro, 233
Lutheran Sailors and Loggers Mission, 183

Madame Damnable's hotel, 37–38, 40, 46, 48
Major, Katharine, 110–11
Malthus, Robert, 70
mandatory reporting requirements, negative effects of, 177
Mannhalt, Guenter, 161
Marble, Luke and Abigail, 30–31
Mark, Mary Ellen, 144–45, 153, 162, 171–73, 175, 178–80
Martin, Joe, 168–69
Maryland: body snatching for medical schools in, 72; public charity recipients in, 18
Mary's Place (organization), 217
Massachusetts: body snatching for medical schools in, 72, 73; care for the poor in, 17; conscription of paupers as sailors in, 18; mental illness treatment in, 21–22; Edward Moore's life in, 30–32; Moore transported back to, 29–30
Matthews, Mark, 106, 112, 122, 134, 136, 137, 161
Maurer, David, 13, 15, 24–25
Maynard, Catherine, 13, 15, 24–25, 34, 40, 44, 54, 56, 59–60, 65
Maynard, David "Doc," 6, 13, 15, 20–21, 24–25, 34, 37–38, 43–45, 53, 57, 59–60, 65
McCall, Cheryl, 145, 162, 172
McCarthy, Mary, 134
McCarty, Clara Antoinette, 56
McDermott, Jim, 168, 180
McDonald, Malcolm, 82, 109
McGowan, Lauren, 204–5
McKechnie, M. E. A., 100–101
McKinney-Vento Homeless Assistance grants, 197–98
Meany, Edmond S., 207
Medicare and Medicaid, 164–65, 233
Medic One system, 167, 186, 199, 206, 216, 222
Mencken, H. L., 210
Mental Health America, 217–18
Mental Health Systems Act of 1980, 155
mental illness: coffeehouse model and, 231; community mental health centers and, 154–55; contract system for treatment of, 22, 57; eugenics movement and, 135; Indigenous peoples' treatment of, 28–29; moral treatment of, 20–21; 19th-century treatment of, 20–24; prevalence in Seattle, 217–18, 228
Mercer, Asa, 147, 210
Merrick, Charles H., 81
Methodist Church, 85
#MeToo movement, 211
Miller, Irene Burns, 140, 202
Miller, William, 208
Minor, T. T., 57

stigma, 121, 124, 170

Street Bean Coffee, 158

Streetwise (documentary), 169, 171–72, 175

Sugg, Nancy, 194

suicide, 31–32, 42, 135, 212

Summers, Lucia, 50

Summers, Robert William, 50, 52

Summerville, Charles, 101

Taft-Hartley Act of 1947, 117

taxation, 92, 217

Taxi Driver (film), 171

temperance movement, 23–24, 40, 134–35

Tent City 1 (Seattle), 194

Tent City 3 (Seattle), 220

Ten-Year Plan to End Homelessness (CEH), 196–97, 200–202, 224

Territorial University of Washington, 56, 77, 147

Theofelis, Jim, 160–61, 177, 180, 195–96, 203

Third Great Awakening, 85

Thompson, R. H., 149

Thorndike (chief of police), 77

Thrush, Coll, 6, 43, 47, 137, 233–34

Train, George Francis, 51

Treaty of Point Elliott (1855), 49

Truman, Harry S., 132

Tucker, John, 68, 78

Tucker, Mary, 68, 78–79

Turner, Frederick Jackson, 36–37, 146, 206–7

Union Gospel Mission, 48

United Way, 216

University District, 8, 166–69, 227, 230–31

University of Washington, 124, 137, 146–47, 166, 169, 230

Urania Cottage (London), 76

Urban Indian Health Institute, 211

US Conference of Mayors, 156

US Department of Housing and Urban Development, 198

US Forest Service, 92

vaccinations, 58–59

Vagabond and Beggars Act of 1494 (England), 15

Venen, Bertha Piper, 52

Verne, Jules, 51

Vietnam War veterans, 152, 153

Volstead Act of 1920, 134

Vol Trumbull, Annette de, 130

Vulcan Corporation, 202

Wald, Lillian, 87, 106, 131, 132

Walker, George, 60

Wappenstein, Charles "Wappy," 106

War on Drugs, 151

War on Poverty, 149

Washington State Medical Society, 98

Washington State Pension Union, 133–34

Way Home Washington, A, 196

Wayside Mission, 83, 96–99, 100–101, 103–4

Wayside Mission Hospital, 106–13, 137

Weed, Gideon A., 58, 98

welfare colonialism, 17, 35